Real Life Diaries

Through the Eyes
of an Eating Disorder

True stories about living with
anorexia nervosa, bulimia
and binge eating disorder

LYNDA CHELDELIN FELL
with
DEBBIE PFIFFNER
JUNE ALEXANDER

FOREWORD BY
JUNE ALEXANDER

TRIGGER WARNING
This book contains potentially distressing content
to readers who live with an eating disorder.
READ WITH CAUTION

Real Life Diaries
Through the Eyes of an Eating Disorder – 1st ed.
True stories about living with anorexia nervosa, bulimia, and binge eating disorder
Lynda Cheldelin Fell/Debbie Pfiffner/June Alexander
Real Life Diaries www.RealLifeDiaries.com

Cover Design by AlyBlue Media, LLC
Interior Design by AlyBlue Media LLC
Published by AlyBlue Media, LLC

ISBN: 978-1-944328-77-1
Library of Congress Control Number: 2016904880
AlyBlue Media, LLC
Ferndale, WA 98248
www.AlyBlueMedia.com

PRINTED IN THE UNITED STATES OF AMERICA

AlyBlue MEDIA

Real Life Diaries

TESTIMONIALS

"CRITICALLY IMPORTANT... I want to say to Lynda that what you are doing is so critically important." –DR. BERNICE A. KING, Daughter of Dr. Martin Luther King

"BRAVE . . . If you do not understand what goes on in the minds of people who have eating disorders, reading *Real Life Diaries: Through The Eyes of an Eating Disorder* will change that. If you feel alone in your own eating disorder but not yet ready to talk about it, the stories in this book will help you see that there are many who suffer like you, and you can get better. If you are an educator, clinician or someone else who wants to better understand eating disorders, the individuals in *Real Life Diaries* tell the straight truth about their thoughts and behaviors, providing a wide variety of ways an eating disorder manages to take hold. The brave individuals who, however painful, share their truth in this book, do it for the benefit of all who are seeking to know the inner world of this devastating and difficult to treat illness." -CAROLYN COSTIN, Founder - Monte Nido Treatment Centers

"INSPIRATIONAL.... Real Life Diaries is the result of heartfelt testimonials from a dedicated and loving group of people. By sharing their stories, the reader will find inspiration and a renewed sense of comfort as they move through their own journey." -CANDACE LIGHTNER, Founder of Mothers Against Drunk Driving

"WONDERFUL...Grief Diaries is a wonderful computation of stories written by the best of experts, the bereaved themselves. Thank you for building awareness about a topic so near and dear to my heart." -DR. HEIDI HORSLEY, Adjunct Professor, School of Social Work, Columbia University, Author, Co-Founder of Open to Hope Organization

"DEEPLY INTIMATE... Grief Diaries is a deeply intimate, authentic collection of narratives that speak to the powerful, often ambiguous, and wide spectrum of emotions that arise from loss. I so appreciate the vulnerability and truth embedded in these stories." -DR. ERICA GOLDBLATT HYATT, Chair of Psychology, Bryn Athyn College

"VITAL... Grief Diaries: Surviving Loss of a Pregnancy gives voice to the thousands of women who face this painful journey every day. Often alone in their time of need, these stories will play a vital role in surrounding each reader with warmth and comfort as they seek understanding and healing in the aftermath of their own loss." -JENNIFER CLARKE, obstetrical R.N., Perinatal Bereavement Committee at AMITA Health Adventist Medical Center

"MOVING... In Grief Diaries, the stories are not only moving but often provide a rich background for any mourner to find a gem of insight that can be used in coping with loss. Reread each story with pen in hand and you will find many that are just right for you." -DR. LOUIS LAGRAND, Author of Healing Grief, Finding Peace

"HEALING... Grief Diaries gives voice to a grief so private, most women bear it alone. These diaries can heal hearts and begin to build community and acceptance to speak the unspeakable. Share this book with your sisters, mothers, grandmothers and friends. Pour a cup of tea together and know that you are no longer alone." -DIANNA VAGIANOS ARMENTROUT, Poetry Therapist & Author of Walking the Labyrinth of My Heart: A Journey of Pregnancy, Grief and Infant Death

"STUNNING... Grief Diaries treats the reader to a rare combination of candor and fragility through the eyes of the bereaved. Delving into the deepest recesses of the heartbroken, the reader easily identifies with the diverse collection of stories and richly colored threads of profound love that create a stunning read full of comfort and hope." -DR. GLORIA HORSLEY, President, Open to Hope Foundation

"HOPE AND HEALING... You are a pioneer in this field and you are breaking the trail for others to find hope and healing." -KRISTI SMITH, Bestselling Author & International Speaker

Through the Eyes of an Eating Disorder

DEDICATION

This book is dedicated to all
who live with an eating disorder.

Through the Eyes of an Eating Disorder

CONTENTS

RESOURCES

Knowledge is a powerful tool in understanding and overcoming an eating disorder. New information is continually emerging. Always hold on to hope and never give up. Following are links to resources:

Academy for Eating Disorders (AED)
www.aedweb.org

Binge Eating Disorder Association
bedaonline.com

Families Empowered and Supporting Treatment of Eating Disorders
(F.E.A.S.T.) – www.feast-ed.org

Gurze/Salucore Eating Disorders Resource Catalog www.edcatalogue.com

National Association of Anorexia Nervosa & Associated Disorders
www.anad.org

National Eating Disorders Association
www.nationaleatingdisorders.org

National Institute of Mental Health
www.nimh.nih.gov/health/topics/eating-disorders/index.shtml

World Eating Disorders Action Day
worldeatingdisordersday.org

BY JUNE ALEXANDER

FOREWORD

An eating disorder is like an uninvited but charismatic invisible guest that develops and embeds in the mind. The longer it stays, the harder it is to budge. It feeds on your sense of self and proceeds to cause a whirlwind of destruction in your life, in your family home, and everywhere you go.

Thank you, Lynda Cheldelin Fell, for creating this opportunity for presenting a fresh perspective, through written narrative, on a deeply challenging and often widely misunderstood illness.

The stories candidly and courageously shared in this volume of the Real Life Diaries series will help to bring home the truth that eating disorders are not a lifestyle choice, a personal weakness, a fad, or a diet gone "too far." The stories show that eating disorders are potentially life-threatening mental and physical illnesses with serious consequences for health, productivity, and relationships.

When a person develops an eating disorder, symptoms manifest around food and often lead to a disconnection between body and self. The person is driven to engage in acts of bodily self-harm rather than self-love. Besides losing their sense of self and identity, the person with the illness often becomes disconnected from others, including family and friends.

For instance, if invited out for dinner with friends, you might avoid and refuse the invitation. Or, if you attend, you spend all your time counting the calories on your plate and calculating how much exercise you must do to appease anxiety and guilt, oblivious to the happy social conversation taking place around the table.

In the United States alone, an estimated twenty million women and ten million men suffer from a clinically significant eating disorder at some time in their life, including anorexia nervosa, bulimia nervosa, binge eating disorder, or other specified feeding or eating disorder (OSFED). Many more people suffer in silence. As highlighted on the inaugural World Eating Disorders Action Day, on June 2, 2016, eating disorders are a global issue.

When one is imprisoned in an eating disorder, grief infiltrates layers of emotion that are numbed and suppressed with thoughts and behaviors of the eating disorder: a constant barrage of guilt, shame, anger, fear, anxiety, sadness, feelings of worthlessness, self-loathing and more. Breaking free from an eating disorder involves re-nourishing the body sufficiently to allow reconnection with healthy thought and behavior patterns. With therapeutic guidance, you then can dig down, tend to, and release pent-up feelings.

When the illness is raging it behaves like a bully in the mind, a bully you cannot see or touch. This bully causes thoughts and behaviors to focus with a magnetic force on food, and rules about food. Initially appearing in the mind as a friend, helping to suppress and appease anxiety, the illness is hellbent on inciting self-deprivation, self-harm and social isolation. In the guise of a coping and managing tool, it separates you from your true sense of self in a subtle, sneaky way that you may be unaware and unable to understand that you are ill. When you do not understand that you are ill, the brain dysfunction caused by the illness convinces you to resist any suggestion of accessing treatment: "I don't need to see a doctor. I'm not sick!"

Denial and concealment of symptoms is a common manifestation of brain changes associated with eating disorders and resulting malnutrition. You may seem a difficult, selfish person when all the time it is the illness making you behave this way. The best hope of avoiding this difficult, alienating and dangerous situation is for early detection and assertive treatment.

The writers in this book are among the many, many people who have missed the small window of opportunity for early intervention. Each has traveled a long and winding road to reach the point where they can reflect, and engage in what is an essential grieving process.

Writing about an experience with an eating disorder can help you to put it in the context of your life, and to see that you are a worthwhile person, deserving of respect, first and foremost—a person who happens to have developed a serious illness. Years lost to illness cannot be reclaimed, but they can be honored and made to count by living life to the full in the present.

The losses involved with an eating disorder can be immense, and affect every aspect of life and, sadly, can culminate in the loss of life itself. The loss of one life is one too many. Losses can start early—I was eleven when my anorexia nervosa developed. Some children are younger than this. Missing out on a normal childhood and adolescence is just the start of a long list of losses. One of the anomalies about an eating disorder is that you can look "normal," maintain top results at school and college, and shine in a high-functioning career, but at great personal cost. This is because part of you is imprisoned in the illness, which saps your confidence, and rules with secrets and shame. You might feel compelled to cling to the eating disorder thoughts and behaviors to get through each day, to manage some control. But the illness is in control; it wants you all to itself. It encourages self-harm because it wants to isolate, debilitate and kill you.

Eating disorders do not affect the mind only. They are also associated with significant physical complications which can affect every major organ in the body, and the mortality rate for people with eating disorders is the highest of all psychiatric illnesses. The illness occurs in both men and women, young and old, rich and poor, and from all cultural backgrounds.

Family and friends may wonder what is happening to you. Often, you have been bright and bubbly, considerate and eager to please; now you are a moody, withdrawn, conflict-charged shadow of yourself. Depending on the nature of the eating disorder, you may have been able to conceal many of the behaviors for years. A person with an eating disorder may go to great lengths to hide, disguise or deny his or her behavior, and fail to recognize that there is anything wrong. However, when you have an eating disorder, the world can become very small and introspective, revolving around issues of weight, shape, eating and body image. One reason an eating disorder is difficult to treat is because its development is an individual and complex pathway, where genetic and personality vulnerabilities interact with social and environmental triggers. However, although a person's genetics may predispose them to developing an eating disorder, this is certainly not the fault of the parents. It is worth noting here that genetics play a role in many illnesses, both mental (for example, schizophrenia) and physical (for example, breast cancer and heart disease). Nobody is to blame. Parents are not to blame when an eating disorder develops but they, together with other family members and friends, can play a crucial role in their loved one's care, support and recovery.

The stories shared here will help you understand that an eating disorder is more than an individual illness; it is a family illness. Everyone in the family is affected in some way and, ideally, everyone will be involved in the recovery process. The benefits of family support are many. However, carers, including parents, partners, friends, grandparents, children and siblings, often also feel distressed, exhausted, confused, anxious, fearful, frustrated, isolated, unhappy, hopeless and powerless. We could equally be presenting a book on eating disorders through the eyes of carers. Importantly, if you have an eating disorder and family of origin support is not available, you can create a family of choice to guide and assist you on the recovery path. Even if you have had an eating disorder for decades, it is possible to recover and live a full life.

I felt delighted and honored when Lynda Cheldelin Fell invited me to write this Foreword. The same year I developed anorexia nervosa, I received a diary for Christmas. I know now that there are only two things to remember in diary keeping: first, date each entry, and second, make no rules. I knew the first rule as a child, but the second one eluded me and deeply affected the story of my life.

The small Christmas gift marked the start of a literary relationship in which the diary would record the loss and recovery of self, and serve as a survival tool in both destructive and constructive ways. The illness, like the diary, thrived on privacy—and encouraged rules and secrets. When I was a child and a young woman, the diary presented as a safe place in which to express and analyze thoughts, and develop coping strategies. But confiding in the diary also strengthened the eating disorder. When rules inevitably were broken, another punishing diet and exercise regime immediately took their place. Nothing was enough, and the rules became secrets within secrets that had to be guarded and hidden from others.

When I eventually reconnected with my authentic self, at age fifty-five, I wrote a memoir, *A Girl Called Tim*. Many readers responded, saying that the sharing of my story had inspired and enabled them to share their story too. This narrative sharing sparked a yearning to go a step farther than the memoir and to explore the role of diary writing in healing from an eating disorder. This has led to the release of *Using Writing as a Therapy for Eating Disorders: The Diary Healer* and participation in the Real Life Diaries series. One of the many benefits of the Real Life Diaries is that participants are encouraged to transition more fully from an "insider" participant to an "outsider" observer of their illness.

Giving people with illness experience a voice, allowing the release of their evidence of lived experience through storytelling and journaling, promotes ongoing healing. It also provides inspiration and gives permission to others to communicate with the narrative and more actively participate in their own healing and recovery. Writing a diary or journal, and sharing a life story in a safe and supportive environment such as the Real Life Diaries, can assist the writer in moving from an inward place of isolation and secrecy to openness, acceptance and acknowledgment of true self.

Personal narratives of illness experience also are gaining recognition as an effective educational and therapeutic tool in addressing and dispelling myths, stigma and shame in the wider community. Presenting the voice of experience in narrative form, besides being cathartic for the writer, can help others to understand what it is like to live with an eating disorder. The patient's narrative, it also is shown, can assist in learning about the effect and effectiveness of therapies and treatments, as well as underlying comorbidity problems such as anxiety, depression, obsessive-compulsive disorder, and substance abuse.

The stories here will take you on a journey within the illness experience. If you identify with any of the symptoms, thoughts or behaviors described, in either yourself or a loved one, explore the resource links on page xi, and reach out for help today.

Don't settle for a part-life. Aim for a full life. You deserve it.

JUNE ALEXANDER
www.junealexander.com
Author of eight books on eating disorders, including *Using Writing as a Therapy for Eating Disorders – The Diary Healer*
(Routledge, London, 2016)

2016 Recipient, Meehan/Hartley Award for Public Service and Advocacy from the Academy for Eating Disorders; Member, World Eating Disorders Action Day 2016 steering committee
References:
www.nedc.com.au | www.feast-ed.org | www.nationaleatingdisorders.org

JUNE 2, 2016
WORLD EATING DISORDERS ACTION DAY
supports the
NINE TRUTHS ABOUT EATING DISORDERS
www.WorldEatingDisordersDay.org
#WeDoAct #WorldEatingDisordersDay

Truth #1: Many people with eating disorders look healthy, yet may be extremely ill.

Truth #2: Families are not to blame, and can be the patients' and providers' best allies in treatment.

Truth #3: An eating disorder diagnosis is a health crisis that disrupts personal and family functioning.

Truth #4: Eating disorders are not choices, but serious biologically influenced illnesses.

Truth #5: Eating disorders affect people of all genders, ages, races, ethnicities, body shapes and weights, sexual orientations, and socioeconomic statuses.

Truth #6: Eating disorders carry an increased risk for both suicide and medical complications.

Truth #7: Genes and environment play important roles in the development of eating disorders.

Truth #8: Genes alone do not predict who will develop eating disorders.

Truth #9: Full recovery from an eating disorder is possible. Early detection and intervention are important.

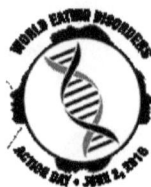

BY LYNDA CHELDELIN FELL

PREFACE

In 1983 a gifted singer by the name of Karen Carpenter died of heart failure at age thirty-two. Not only did her death shock the nation, the cause of her heart failure from complications of anorexia nervosa brought a little-known eating disorder into the public spotlight. I was seventeen at the time, and I mourned alongside fans around the world. But I had never heard of anorexia nervosa, and couldn't fathom what would cause such a famous singer at the height of her career to starve herself literally to death.

Karen's anorexia led the way to increased visibility and awareness about eating disorders. Yet in the decades since her death, research continues to be underfunded, insurance coverage for treatment is inadequate, and societal acceptance of different body sizes remains unchanged.

I live with an eating disorder on the opposite end of the spectrum: binge eating disorder. Shrouded in secrecy and shame, my eating habits led to severe obesity. Not only was I too embarrassed to seek help, I dreaded going to the doctor for any reason. Why? Because at the beginning of every visit the nurse charted my weight on the scale. I didn't own a scale at home, making it easy to lie to myself. But the clinic scale was the moment of truth, a reality I found too hard to face.

Ten years ago, I turned forty years old. But I felt like I was ninety. My knees hurt, I was easily winded, and wore size 22. Afraid of the future, I became determined to regain control of my health—and my life. I shed exactly one hundred pounds through healthy eating and daily walking. I finally succeeded at gaining control over my binge eating illness.

Along the way, I also discovered that helping others was a powerful way to heal my own heart. The Grief Diaries and Real Life Diaries series was born and built on this belief. By writing books narrating our journeys through life's experiences, our written words become a portable support group for others. When we swap stories, we feel less alone. It is comforting to know someone else understands the shoes we walk in, and the challenges we face along the way.

Real Life Diaries: Through the Eyes of an Eating Disorder is an inside look at the world through the eyes of those who live with anorexia nervosa, bulimia, and binge eating. The collection of stories will shed critical insight into such an illness, and comfort those who share the path by helping them understand that they aren't alone on the journey. If you struggle with an eating disorder, the following true stories are written by courageous women who know exactly how you feel, for they've been in your shoes and have walked the same path. Perhaps the shoes are a different size or style, but may you find comfort in these stories and the understanding that you aren't truly alone on the journey. For we walk ahead, behind, and right beside you.

Wishing you healing and hope from the Diaries village.

Warm regards,

Lynda Cheldelin Fell

CHAPTER ONE

The Beginning

The thing that is really hard, and really amazing, is
giving up on being perfect and beginning the work
of becoming yourself. - ANNA QUINDLEN

Where do eating disorders begin? Are we born with it? Does it develop out of learned behavior? In years past, it was once considered a lifestyle choice. Today, eating disorders are recognized as serious illnesses defined as anorexia nervosa, bulimia nervosa, and binge eating disorder. Because each journey is as unique as a fingerprint, in this chapter each writer shares the beginning of her story to help you understand the perspectives throughout this book.

*

JUNE ALEXANDER
June is a 65-year-old living
beyond anorexia nervosa

I am a Baby Boomer, born between Christmas and New Year's Eve 1950. I lived with my parents, sister and paternal grandparents on a dairy farm, at the head of a beautiful, fertile river valley in Victoria, Australia. The property was adjacent to what is now called Mitchell River National Park. This bushland would become my playground, my escape, my soul-place, and the place from which I would draw strength in the decades to follow.

At the time I was born, my parents did not own a car—my dad was still using draft horses to cultivate his fields—but Grandpa had a Ford, and this vehicle provided transport to the nearest hospital at Bairnsdale, a town twenty miles away, for my birth. My mother had been to the doctor the day before and was told to return in three weeks for another checkup. She went home. I was born six weeks prematurely, the very next day.

During this period the family home was not connected to electricity and had no running hot water. Communication with life outside the valley was provided by a large wireless radio that sat on the kitchen floor, a phone that was fixed to the passage wall, and weekly newspapers. My sister was thirty months older. Photographs taken during our childhood show my sister in pink, with her long brown hair in ringlets, and me in blue, with snowy hair cropped short.

My mother called me Tim when I was good and Toby when I was bad. I was happy as a tomboy. I loved helping Dad on the farm. I did chores from age five, filling kerosene bottles for the lamps at night, feeding the chooks, collecting the hen eggs, and feeding the calves at the dairy. I glowed with pride when Dad told an uncle that although I was a left-hander, I was his righthand man.

My greatest interest inside the home was reading and writing. The written word somehow seemed safe. It seemed precious. I don't recall my parents ever reading to me, and I never saw either of them reading a book, but nonetheless I had this passion for reading and writing, along with an affinity for nature.

Two big events occurred at age five. My formal education began in a one-room, twenty-pupil school that was surrounded by crops and cow-studded fields. To get there I pedaled a bike two and a half miles. The same year, my dad bought his first car, and my grandparents moved into a house in Bairnsdale. Grandma died when I was ten. I missed her and spoke with her in my prayers, whispering under the blankets each night, long after the candle was snuffed out. When Grandma and Grandpa lived on the farm, I sometimes awoke next morning in their bed, feeling safe and snug with a grandparent on either side. My parents would place me there in the middle of the night when my bed was needed for visitors. Before getting up, Grandma would let me lie close to her for a while, and would gently scratch my back; she would let me help clip up her tight-fitting corsets, and brush her beautiful, long silvery-white hair which she wore pinned into a neat bun during the day. She also taught me to knit and crochet. The only intimacy I recall as a child was this time with my grandma.

When Grandma died she left a small glass jar with a handwritten piece of scrap paper taped on top of the lid, stating "This is June's." The jar contained pennies, halfpennies, threepences and sixpences. I treasured that little jar, for its message more than its contents. In years to come, those three words, which I still have, penned in my grandma's hand, would give me strength.

Meanwhile my love of words continued. At age eight I wanted to be an author. Books, at home and at school, whether age-appropriate or not, fired my imagination. At age nine I won my first prize, a pen, in a story-writing competition. Until this time, I had only one teacher, who took all six grades in the school. Then a new teacher came. He was a cousin, just out of teachers' college, and he boarded in our home. My sister and I found him creepy.

My sister and I shared a bedroom, which had a fireplace and a tall sash window. Before getting into bed, my sister had various routines, one of which was to look in the wardrobe, under our beds, and up the fireplace chimney. She refused to tell me what she was looking for. Some nights while lying in bed, she insisted there was a light outside the window. Unable to placate her, I would get out of bed and assure her there was no light. But she insisted to the point where I also would get upset, and call our parents in. I tried to be helpful and well-behaved to compensate for the disturbances caused by my sister's confusing behaviors.

Helping Dad on the farm was one way to avoid being inside with my mother and sister, who seemed to argue a lot, but also needed each other in a way I didn't understand. They called me stubborn and pigheaded for preferring to help Dad or to wander alone in the bush, rather than stay inside or play at a friend's house.

In sixth grade, the final year of primary school, my world changed. Two weeks after my eleventh birthday, in the summer holidays of 1962, I got my first period. I had watched bulls mating with cows plenty of times, but was completely unaware of human habits.

When Mum noticed blood in my bed one morning, she pulled me aside and gave a brief description. I felt my world had fallen in. For a week every month I would have that bleeding; every month, because I was a girl. I didn't want to be a girl; I wanted to be Tim. I felt mortified and hoped Dad would not notice there was something different about me. Several weeks later the new school year started.

I was the only girl in the school with breasts. When I ran, they bounced up and down and hurt. If I held them they didn't hurt, but this was embarrassing to do when playing with the boys or within sight of my schoolteacher cousin. The following month the teacher announced that the school doctor, who did health checks every three or four years, would visit in June. We were given consent forms to take home. I became very nervous at the thought of needing to undress when the doctor came; his visit was only three months away and there didn't seem any way out. Then one day the tension suddenly eased. I had no idea, of course, that anorexia nervosa was developing. I began to eat less and exercise more. The school doctor came and went, but I remained too afraid to eat. My periods ceased. My ankles swelled, sores broke out on my fingers, I ran instead of walked, even in the rain. My parents despaired. A major concern was "What will people think?"

Communication with the wider world took a step forward when our family homestead was connected to electricity, and we got a television set. But I couldn't feel excited because, well, I could not sit still to watch television. A Christmas gift of a small diary, however, did excite me—we bonded immediately.

*

OLIVIA ANTHONY
Olivia is a 44-year-old living
with anorexia and bulimia

My eating disorder began when I was about thirteen. I guess I would say it was a slippery slope time for me. It was a time when I had my first boyfriend. We mostly just talked on the phone, since I wasn't allowed to date yet. Like most of the people on my dad's side of the family, I was naturally thin—underweight, in fact. My mom often made disparaging comments about her own body, wishing she was thin. My dad was always taking food away from her and telling her to lose weight. I remember him telling me once that I had better be careful so I wouldn't get fat. I started thinking that I better never let myself get fat or he won't love me or be proud of me. Also during this time, I suffered from obsessive-compulsive disorder. I didn't know that was the term for it until many years later. That, for me, was most distressing. I felt like I had to touch things over and over again to prevent my mom from dying. I felt crazy. I would, for example, turn the light on, then I had to go back and touch the light switch again. And again. Over and over.

My mom took a trip to California with a friend and I was so sad and worried about her. I worried about something happening to her. It was really stressful for me. I don't even remember how long she was gone. Probably just a week. I felt like my world was out of control. Anything could happen to her and then I would be motherless. That terrified me. It wasn't until I started high school where my eating disorder eclipsed my obsessive-compulsive disorder. I was an athlete and felt so proud of myself for having only an orange for breakfast and restricting food all day, even with a vigorous volleyball practice. However, I was able to avoid really falling hard into the trap of anorexia until my freshman year of college. That's when I fully became sick and entrenched in anorexia's grasp. My roommate and I ate mostly hot cereal for every meal. I remember doing calorie calculations during class. I set a goal of not going over a certain number of calories. On top of that, I started getting up at 5 a.m. to work out. I also ran at lunch and when classes were done in the afternoon. Then my roommate and I walked in the evenings. At the end of that school year I moved back home. I distinctly remember thinking how I would focus on staying thin and working. Food, weight, and working out consumed my thoughts.

*

CHRISTINE BASTONE
Christine is a 49-year-old living
with binge eating disorder

I have always liked to eat. I have never been one of those girls who picks at her food, or eats only salad. Even so, I was skinny until my early twenties. My eating disorder started while I was going through my divorce back in 1991. That was the first time I had lived alone. Since I did live alone, I could indulge in all the food I wanted.

I think it came on a little more gradually than it sounds. It may have started with little things, like when I was in high school I started using my own money to buy the yummy ice cream that was on the a la carte menu. I bought candy at the local five-and-dime store with my own money too. I started eating at night when the rest of my family was on vacation and I had the house to myself. Little by little my problem grew, until now it is huge and very much out of control.

While I absolutely hate diets, I have tried them a few times. The one I remember most occurred in 1994. I was in a weight-loss support group at my church. We met weekly, and there were three books about the program. This is when I first tried low-fat foods from the grocery store. I did lose some weight doing that. But I still needed to lose more when it either ended or I moved from Ohio to Florida in 1995. Otherwise, I have tried approaches more than diets, usually from books. *When You Eat at the Refrigerator, Pull Up a Chair* by Geneen Roth, *French Women Don't Get Fat* by Mireille Guiliano, and *I Can Make You Thin* by Paul McKenna are three that stand out. I like Paul McKenna the best, and will talk more about him later.

I have tried to limit my carbs without much success, as I love them more than any other food! And I also tried to limit my fat. I found Susan Powter to be absolutely fascinating when I saw her on TV, and in her book *Stop The Insanity*. These days I'm not interested in any actual diet, and I know that any harsh or punishing method is not going to work for me. I gravitate to gentler approaches. But right now I am absolutely miserable and disgusted. I cannot stop bingeing. My emotional hunger is sky-high, and I constantly try to fill it with food. I am probably at my highest weight ever. While I rarely stuff myself anymore, I frequently eat until I am really full. And I feel quite powerless to stop any of it.

*

LISA BRUNS
Lisa is a 52-year-old living
with binge eating disorder

I remember being obese at a very young age. My mother would try to put me on diets. Coming from a poor family, I ate a lot of Mexican food, and it was just unhealthy. I cried all the time because I had no control over my eating.

*

LYNDA CHELDELIN FELL
Lynda is a 50-year-old living
with binge eating disorder

It's hard to know when my binge eating began. I've always loved food. I'm the fourth of five kids, and my mom is a good cook. As a family, we sat down to dinner every night when Dad got home from work. I enjoyed Mom's savory meal but then shortly after clearing the dinner dishes would make lemon bars or chocolate chip cookies. I rarely experience satiety, the physical sensation of feeling full. So eating half a batch of lemon bars or three pieces of cake in the evening after a full dinner wasn't uncomfortable.

As a teenager, my older sister and I often visited the library and then bought snacks on the way home. We sat in the living room reading our library books while munching on the snacks tucked beside us. My sister often went for sunflower seeds, but my weakness was candy, especially chocolate. I could eat an entire bag of candy in one sitting. I wasn't heavy. At five feet five inches, I wore size twelve jeans which, at the time, was considered average. But my mother was very conscious of her figure, and those of her four daughters. She was always dieting, and so were we. But diets never lasted long in our house. I was most happy when creating confections in the kitchen, and even happier eating them.

But that all changed when I became pregnant with my firstborn. I remember feeling like sky's the limit on what I could eat. Maternity clothing would hide everything! I gained forty pounds during my first pregnancy, but my eating didn't slow down after giving birth. I ate a pint of Baskin-Robbins ice cream every night. If you bought seven pints, your eighth one was free. I earned a lot of free pints.

Over the next ten years, I happily birthed three more babies. And my weight spiraled out of control. I managed to lose a large amount of weight a number of times. I loved how I looked when thin, but maintaining that weight loss was a struggle. I had to be extra strict. I couldn't eat just one nibble. Like a magician, I could make a batch of brownies disappear within short order. In addition, I lacked satiety; my stomach never registered full. I didn't know this wasn't normal. Each evening when I brought out the ice cream and offered my husband a bowl, he declined, saying he was still full from dinner. I couldn't understand such a notion.

I never ate three meals a day. Instead, I preferred to graze all day long. And my food choices were terrible. I cooked a hot dinner for my family just like my mom did, but I never ate the vegetables unless they were smothered in cheese sauce or garlic butter. Why bother? To my thinking, they offered calories that were better spent on comfort food waiting for me after the dinner dishes were done.

Once the kids were old enough to notice that a freshly baked batch of cookies had mysteriously disappeared, I began to feel guilty. But I also got crafty at hiding my problem. I never owned up to eating an entire batch of lemon bars in one sitting; I was terribly embarrassed at my lack of control. I never sought treatment for binge eating because it wasn't until years later that I realized I even had a disorder. It simply wasn't discussed, and food was something my large family enjoyed.

As a yo-yo dieter, I hated going out in public unless I was thin. As a large woman, I noticed that in general, society ignores obese people. We are invisible or dismissed. I readily smile at strangers, but when I was obese, that smile was rarely reciprocated. When I was thin, smiles were abundantly exchanged. Why are we judged on size alone? I had a kind, compassionate heart. I had good manners. I was intelligent. I was a good mother and good wife. I wasn't sloppy or lazy. My clothing was clean, and I showered daily. Yet I couldn't deny that the difference of how I was treated was based solely on my body's size.

The pivotal moment came ten years ago, when I turned forty. As an obese woman, I avoided healthcare unless it was something urgent. But I worked in the medical field, and my annual exam was long overdue. I knew it was probably time to schedule an appointment, which I did. I was sitting in the reception area of the doctor's office when the nurse finally called my name. I felt like I was walking a pirate's plank as I followed the nurse to the scale. I set my purse down, took off my coat, removed my shoes and anything else that might possibly add weight. And the moment came. I stood on the scale and waited. The nurse didn't flinch as she wrote down my weight. But I had sticker shock: I weighed a whopping xxx pounds. How did I not know I had gotten that large?

It was as if a light switch flipped somewhere in a far recess of my brain. From that moment forward, I started walking. My neighbor joined me. She had a puppy that needed exercise, and I was determined to overcome my weight before the damage to my body advanced beyond repair. So off me and my neighbor went every morning like clockwork. We walked my kids to the bus stop, and when the bus pulled away we continued on to the nearby cemetery that offered flat pathways, scenic trees, and a peaceful ambiance. Every morning, Monday through Friday, we walked an average of two to three miles. I also changed my diet. I didn't weigh portions; I didn't count calories, because that hadn't worked in the past. My only diet rule was that whatever I put into my mouth had to be nourishing; it had to be useful to my body. If it came from a box or a can, I knew the artificial additives canceled out most nutritional value. This meant that processed food of any kind was not only on the naughty list, but much of it was downright harmful. At first everything tasted bland and boring. Carrots and celery were considered rabbit food, and I missed the satiny texture of rich chocolate ganache. But I remained determined. Much to my delight, my taste buds recalibrated and healthy food actually began tasting good. Who knew?!

Since I didn't own a scale, on the first of the month my neighbor brought her scale to the top of the driveway so we could check my progress. Between the morning walks and my eating for health, I lost steady weight every month. I didn't have a set weight I wanted to reach. My goal was to get healthy, not wear a bikini. But one day the scale revealed a triumph that my neighbor and I never expected—I had shed one hundred pounds.

Ten years later, I've kept the weight off. Has it been easy? Some days, yes. Some days, no. Stress, hormones and lack of sleep are big triggers for me. So I have to remain vigilant, because for a binge eater, all it takes is one sinful nibble and down the rabbit hole I go.

*

JUSTINE HILDEN
Justine is a 27-year-old living
with binge eating disorder

I grew up in a loving and supportive home. I was a happy person growing up. I have struggled with perfectionism and anxiety since I was just a few years old. I think that was the original trigger, just waiting to be pulled when the time was right. In high school I had friends who struggled with anorexia and bulimia. I remember thinking, "What is their problem?" "Why are they doing this to themselves?" "Don't they see they are perfect the way they are?" I also remember thinking, "That will never be me."

When I graduated high school I was happy, having a great group of friends, working a job I enjoyed, and enjoying time with my great family. I enjoyed my summer, relaxing, being active, going camping, and spending time up north. In the back of my mind, I kept thinking about the summer coming to an end and that I would be moving to attend the University of Minnesota-Duluth for my freshman year of college. I had never been away from home. When the time came, I was a wreck. So many girls were moving in, so excited to be getting away from home, starting out on their own, and here I was lying in my bed, sobbing. This lasted for months. I cried, slept, and tried to go to class. I am one who, even in the most stressful and hardest times, pushes through what I need to do, and that was to go to class and get good grades. In between, I would sleep and cry. This led me to a deep depression, a sadness and loneliness that I had never felt before. My roommate, who knew me prior to college, would point out how tough it was to live with me in my current state. Let me tell you, she was a trouper and a great support throughout all of freshman year. But, back to the depression, a professor recognized that I was really struggling. She recommended that I see an on-campus counselor. At first I thought she was crazy, or that I was. I had never seen a therapist, and was scared to. But I did it, and am so grateful for my teacher and counselor. I needed that professional to talk to.

I made it through my freshman year. I gained an excessive amount of weight, which I attributed to college life. A friend, whom I met in my freshman year, and I decided to begin a diet program the summer before sophomore year. I followed it strictly, and lost the weight I had gained. I felt pretty good about myself. I felt happy with where I was both physically and mentally. But then sophomore year started, and for some reason I thought I could handle another year in Duluth. I had ups and downs, continued to see my therapist, and really struggled. After the strict "dieting" over the summer, I decided I "deserved" to eat, and that's what I did. It became like freshman year all over again. My weight just went up and up. I decided Duluth wasn't for me after a year and a half of struggle, and I moved back home in December 2007 to attend Bethel University. I thought things would just go back to normal, and that I would be happy just because I was back at home.

Well that's not how it went. The transition to a new school, the stress of the academics and the stress of meeting new people, took a toll, and I continued in my spiral of depression. I had gained some weight, and it continued to go up, gradually for a while, though. It started off slowly, a few pounds here, a few pounds there. But it all started to add up. Throughout 2008, I gained a significant amount of weight, and I was heavier than before. So I tried more dieting. This time I chose shakes, because then I wouldn't have to think so much about the food I was eating, and the planning. I lost some weight. Still, I had no idea that what I was dealing with was an eating disorder, so bear with me. During spring 2009, my mom and I decided to see a doctor to see what I was dealing with. Maybe it was my thyroid, or so we guessed. Everything came back fine. I thought, "I'm not fine, this is not normal. What is wrong with me?" I started to binge eat and then purge. I did the purging thing for about a month. Then it just became bingeing and overeating. I knew these things were not okay. I knew this all too well in high school with one of my best friends. But I only knew about bulimia and anorexia. I wasn't thin; I was gaining weight, not losing.

I got online and googled. I wanted to know if there was a name for what I was dealing with. I started reading up on it. I remember showing my mom what came up on binge eating and compulsive overeating, and told her, "I think I know what's wrong with me." I saw my regular physician again, and she recommended that I seek treatment through The Emily Program in St. Paul. In June 2009, that's what I did.

Looking back, I thought there would be a quick fix. And I was doing it for my mom, who was stressed with my weight gain, not so much for me. I went weekly, seeing a therapist and dietitian. I didn't work hard; I didn't really even try. I would go through the motions of going to treatment. They told me what to work on, I would nod my head, agree with what they said, and go back to my ways when I left. After six months I decided I didn't need help. I told myself that I wasn't crazy and could figure it out on my own.

The year 2010 didn't get any better. I was using food to cope with getting through my senior year of college and gaining weight. Dieting couldn't help because I wanted food, I needed food. After gaining more weight, and graduating from college in December of that year, I decided to try The Emily Program again. This time it was my decision and mine alone. I knew I needed to be there. I knew I needed help.

I began there in January 2011 and have been there ever since. I started out in weekly individual therapy and saw a dietitian. They referred me to intensive outpatient therapy, three days a week. The first few weeks were tough. I thought everyone else in the group was nuts and that I was normal. The rituals and thoughts they had around food were crazy. But the more I was there, and the more I let myself explore who I was and what I was struggling with, and the more I was willing to be open, I found out that I had some serious issues not only with food, but also with relationships, self-esteem, and self-worth. In the fall of 2011, I got my first teaching job as a special education teacher. Everything seemed to be falling into place. It ended up being a very unsupportive and unhealthy work environment. My eating disorder only escalated, and my self-worth plummeted. I considered never teaching again, which caused a lot of stress in itself, because being a teacher was all I ever knew and wanted since I was just a little girl. I resigned from that position and decided to take care of myself. I continued at The Emily Program, but had stepped down from the Intensive Program when my job got to be too much. The intensive outpatient program was by far the most challenging time of my life, but I learned so much and grew so much in the time that I did it.

I got a new job in January 2012. I have had my ups and downs, the stresses of teaching special education, the loss of my grandma, losing my childhood pets, stress with relationships, specifically with my mom, and just the stress of being an adult. A big challenge began when my dietitian of four years moved out of state to a different Emily Program location. He changed my life, and I want to keep working at this and prove I can do this. I learned so much from him. He left in the fall of 2015. I ate and gained weight that I have since lost through normalizing my relationship with food. Therefore I continue to struggle. When things are tough, I still use food, but not always. When I do, I can recognize it, which I couldn't do before. I am not yet in recovery. I am not sure what recovery will look like for me, but I do know that I am headed there.

*

LYDIA KENYON
Lydia is a 22-year-old living
with anorexia nervosa

My eating disorder began when I hit puberty and was too afraid to ask anyone for help. Stuck on my own, I had miserable monthly cycles and began to look for a way to change that. Through reading teen magazines, I found out that some women athletes cease menstruating because of their rigorous exercise routines. So I began to exercise more and look into healthier food options. What could have been a partially healthy thing spiraled into a disaster, and I found myself in the throes of a restrictive eating disorder at the age of thirteen. For many years I let my eating disorder ruin my life and control everything. I was in and out of treatment, mostly to appease my parents. Then in September 2015, I knew something had to change. My marriage was a shambles, my emotions were always on edge, and I was so tired. I began to see a dietitian that I had worked with a few years previously and she helped me put together a treatment team at the hospital in my small hometown. Since the first day I met with her, things have been looking up. Recovery is the best decision I have made in my life so far. I just hope and pray that I have the strength to continue in it.

*

REBEKKAH KOONS
Rebekkah is a 29-year-old living with
an eating disorder not otherwise specified

If someone were to sit me down and say, "Rebekkah, when did you decide it was a good idea to start starving yourself?" I would have no answer. In my senior year of high school, I decided to go back to a public school. I was hoping that this time I wouldn't be bullied like I had been in seventh grade when I had to go to a small private school. I had the nicest car at school, and grew from a girl who didn't fit into her own skin into one with long legs and blonde hair. Halfway through my year, I picked up smoking to go along with my new image, and lost a little weight. I never thought about my weight before. I was always tall and skinny and was on the gymnastics team earlier and never once thought about how I looked. I think it was the comments I received from people that opened my eyes. I suffered a traumatic eye injury when I was five and ended up having nine operations. That led to being bullied my whole life because of how it looked. Suddenly people were throwing compliments at me. What was this? I didn't know it at the time, but I had an obsessive personality. Once my mind got fixated on something, I had to know every detail and roll it over and over in my mind for weeks, months, or sometimes years. I started analyzing my body and comparing myself to other girls, and thought that skinny just looked better.

A short time after I graduated, a girl was in the office and pointed to her computer. "Look at this site. This girl is all upset over a slice of pizza. This site is disgusting," she said. I looked over her shoulder. There were pictures of thin girls and various accounts on what they ate and didn't eat, and unfamiliar words like Ana and Ed. Something flipped in my brain, just like a light switch. *Click.* I was obsessed. I secretly found the site, joined it and read almost every blog. I felt peace. I found a place where I belonged. All my stresses from the day, anything bad that would happen, it was okay because I had this site.

I moved to England after that year, and that's when things spiraled completely out of control. I was living in a flat with an overweight girl who hated me. I had no transportation or money, and I spent all my volunteering hours at work on the blogsite, because I was incredibly lonely. Secretly, I bought every book I could find on eating disorders. I decided my extra spending money was better spent on books than food. I watched every documentary I could, and engrossed myself completely into this new world so I didn't have to participate in my own.

I wasn't losing any weight, though. I didn't understand. I was doing everything my online friends told me to: drinking lots of peppermint tea when I felt hungry, and chewing and spitting food so I could taste it but not swallow it. I chugged water before bed so that when I woke up and went to the bathroom, I would feel lighter. I walked to church on Sundays and then I would come home and make a huge bowl of pasta and eat it all. I stopped smoking, as we weren't allowed to. I had exactly seven cigarettes I brought with me, hardly enough to lose any weight.

Soon it was time to go tour Europe by myself for two weeks. I went to London and had drinks in the hotel lounge and went to see the "The Phantom of the Opera." I took a train to Paris and stayed across from the Louvre and spent two whole days exploring every inch of the place. I went to the beautiful city of Venice, and then to Rome. I didn't think about my weight; I was busy exploring and being by myself, wondering if I'd get lost or kidnapped, but I was not counting calories. When I got back home to the States, I realized that with all that walking I had finally lost some weight. I started smoking again and began a new job at the hospital.

There was a new shift, and my obsession got to its highest. I chain-smoked in my new apartment and lived on pop ice. While working the second shift, I ate something small for dinner in the cafeteria before going home to smoke, eat the ice, and sleep. I went from xxx straight down to xxx pounds. I saw my doctor, because there was also something very strange about my eating disorder. I wanted to keep my secret at all cost, while at the same time I wanted someone to know. Someone to help. I reached out to my primary doctor, who had an eating disorder, and she referred me to a counselor. I liked the counselor for a little while. I remember it was raining one morning as I drove downtown to one of my sessions. My counselor worked in a beautiful brick building, and as I arrived I thought, "I made it. I am just as strong as any of those girls on the websites. I am skinnier and stronger than they are." I turned my car around and never saw that counselor again.

It was my father's death a while later, when I was in North Carolina chasing after a boy, that really put me back over the edge. Now that I had gotten to such a low weight, any weight I gained at all I literally felt I could feel. I knew that people worried about me, but it made me smile that I could do what so few people couldn't. I also used starving as my coping mechanism. With my father's death, I lost five pounds. Someone looks at me wrong, lose another pound, and so on. This continued until my obsession started to slowly turn to something else: drinking. Drinking meant calories, but I didn't care. I gained weight back, got my own apartment, and secluded myself from people. It really didn't bother me a bit.

I no longer drink and currently live with my boyfriend. I constantly try to keep busy so I don't sink into that obsession again. It'll never go away, I'll always have the scars and I'll always carry around the thoughts. It's scary to know that it could happen again, and even though I didn't take the route of getting help or going to a treatment center, I was able to save myself. That thought reassures me that if I again become obsessed, I can save myself.

*

RUTH PAPALAS
Ruth is a 58-year-old living
with binge eating disorder

I wish I were as fat as the first time I *thought* I was fat. When I was around thirteen or fourteen, an older girl at church poked me in the belly and told me I'd better lose that, or I was going to be fat forever. I was only slightly overweight. I had boyfriends, and I didn't give much thought to what she said. I didn't believe her until I was around eighteen, and it started to look like she was right.

There were five of us kids in the family. Whatever was put on the table is what we ate. If we didn't eat dinner, we didn't get dessert. I loved desserts. When Mom and Dad took us out to eat, we had to eat everything we ordered, because they paid for it. We had to get our money's worth. When we went to a buffet, we really got our money's worth. When I started working in restaurants and we got an employee discount, I got my money's worth. When I went to college the first time, I stayed only for six months. During that time, I probably gained the "freshman fifteen" plus ten more. The food was not good there, and we ordered lots of pizza. We figured out how to cook food in a popcorn maker in our room. We got care packages with food from home. I ate. When I returned home, I went back to working in a restaurant. I dieted off and on after college. I tried Slim-Fast, over-the-counter diet pills, a doctor who gave me shots, etc. Then I found a doctor who would prescribe "black beauties" or "speed." The cool thing was that my insurance paid for most of the prescription. I lost a lot of weight! I looked great. After the doctor was arrested, that ended.

I married. We ate out a lot, and the weight piled on. Then I got pregnant. I had toxemia, but I didn't know it. I really gained weight. My husband voiced his negative opinion of me and my weight loud and clear. His attitude did not help me lose weight. In fact, after I tried to lose weight and lost fifteen or twenty pounds, I thought I was looking pretty good. Better, anyway. He said it didn't help. I gained more. Nerves? Stress? We divorced. I remarried, to a man who thought and still thinks I'm beautiful.

In time, I found a chiropractor who also counseled people who needed to lose weight. He told me that my body was not using carbohydrates. Every time I ate bread or cake or pasta, it was going directly to my hips. He gave me a low carb diet, which I followed for a while. I lost about fifty pounds. After a few months I missed bread, cake, and pasta and started eating it all again. I regained all I had lost and then some. My legs, back, and feet hurt all the time. I read books, followed diets like Fit for Life and low carb diets, and journaled, but I just loved to eat. I had been to my family doctor and diet doctors who I thought could help me. I was looking for a magic pill or cure—anything. I found that I eat when I'm hungry, by myself or with people, sad, happy, and satiated. I am an emotional eater and I'm full of emotions. I'm always feeling something, so I'm always eating something. Emotional eating is the way I cope and/or avoid feelings. Unmet needs drive me to emotional eating, which leads to bingeing. It's a vicious cycle. My dad had a heart attack and was in the hospital. While he was in intensive care, I found myself in the emergency room receiving a breathing treatment, I knew I was in trouble. My dad died from the heart attack a week or so later.

I started having an annoying cough. I coughed even if I walked short distances. Someone anonymously slipped a brochure about asthma onto my desk. I read it and sought out my family doctor. He sent me to a lung specialist, a pulmonologist, who diagnosed me with asthma. When he inquired about my family history, he asked if my dad was still living. I said no. He asked, "Heart attack?" Shortly after that I picked up a Women's World Magazine with an article about gastric bypass surgery. I started researching gastric bypass, mortality rates, and the best doctors and hospitals. I learned that I could easily find myself having a heart attack or developing diabetes if I continued on the path I was on. I made an appointment to go to a seminar. Then I had an appointment with the doctor and scheduled surgery.

My family was not in favor of my having the gastric bypass. My family doctor was also not in favor. My pulmonologist said, "This surgery will probably save your life." My sympathetic husband said, "If you live through the surgery, maybe I'll consider it." He had the same surgery one year later. Some people thought that was the easy way out. For me it was the only way out. Gastric bypass surgery is not easy. Laparoscopic surgery was not available to me at the time I had the gastric bypass. I had an open Roux-En-Y surgery. It was painful. I lost over one hundred pounds. I went from a size xxx to a size xxx. That's the lowest I got.

There are rules that go with a gastric bypass. There are things you should eat and things you should avoid. At first I followed the rules. The pouch worked. Then I found that I actually could eat some candy and cookies and drink during meals and I didn't get sick. I tried other old favorites. Some things I could eat, some I could not. I thought I was safe. After all, I had had a gastric bypass. I'm still an emotional eater (which leads me to bingeing) and I'm still full of emotions. I've read that I'm one of those people who "eat" their emotions. I have gained back about xxx pounds and crept up to a size xxx. I'm sick of myself. I'm sick of the extra weight. I can't understand how I can control most other things in my life, but not my weight.

*

DEBBIE PFIFFNER
Debbie is a 56-year-old living
with anorexia nervosa

My eating disorder, anorexia nervosa, began rearing its ugly head when I was seventeen years old. As a child I was neither overweight or underweight, just a child of average weight. The summer prior to starting high school, at the age of fourteen, my body changed. I was always tall, taller than most of the kids in my class. But that summer I grew to my full height of five feet nine and a half inches, and my body thinned out to around xxx pounds. I was constantly being told how thin I looked, and I began to love the compliments and felt really good about my body. As I continued through high school, the regular teenage problems and angst caused me to gain some weight. About xxx pounds. Even at xxx pounds and five feet nine and a half inches, I was not considered overweight. But the compliments stopped coming.

During the summer between my junior and senior years, my sister had her first baby at age eighteen. It was an exciting time for her and also an exciting time for me. I got to help with her new baby. As my senior year progressed, between my job, schoolwork, and spending as much time as I could with my sister and her new baby, I began to miss meals, and eating less and less when I finally did eat.

The less I ate, the thinner I got. The compliments started coming again, and I now supplemented the not eating with exercising and running every day. Then the compliments turned into "You're way too thin!" To a person suffering from anorexia, that is the best compliment you can give.

Throughout the year, my family and friends started to voice their concerns. Although I knew the scale was going down at a fast pace, I still thought I was doing okay. I was skinny! What could be better? As the years went by and the scale read xxx pounds, I started to understand that something was not right. I just didn't know what. One day I was soaking in the tub filled with hot water just to stay warm. Someone left a copy of an old Reader's Digest near the tub. I picked it up and started to page through it. I stopped when I came to an article on a new disease affecting young women that affects both physical and mental health. That disease was anorexia nervosa. I now knew exactly what was wrong with me. This article was about me!

I showed the article to my sister. Then my parents became involved. I was sent to the doctor and then put in the hospital where they brought me trays of food, which of course I couldn't eat. That caused them to bring more food. It was an endless battle.

I remember my parents arguing. Everyone was frustrated. I was sent to a new doctor, hospitalized and again given food, vitamins and supplements. They had me see a psychiatrist, a psychologist, a dietitian, and even attend group therapy in the hospital's psychiatric ward. But no one understood. No one could fathom why I refused to eat. What they didn't understand was that I was not refusing to eat; I was beyond that. I literally could not force myself to eat. The anxiety surrounding every morsel of food that went into my mouth was unbearable. This was the late 1970s and early 1980s. Eating disorders were not common. Most people, even professionals, were unaware of this disease and did not know how to treat it. They thought appetite stimulants and supplements forced upon me were the answer. Of course they weren't. And the more they pushed, the harder I pushed back, eventually just walking away.

There were more months of suffering, of lying awake at night because I was afraid that if I fell asleep I would die. One Christmas, I remember my dad telling everyone to be extra nice to me because this was probably going to be the last Christmas I would be with them. Then one day, sick, weak, and tired of it all, I went to my refrigerator and proceeded to eat everything I could find. Of course this resulted in my getting very sick. But once I started eating, I couldn't stop.

For about a year I ate with abandon. I tripled my body weight. Of course I was miserable, but I couldn't stop it. Then, without even realizing it, things started to change. I found myself just eating when I was hungry, and the excess body weight began to come off. About a year later I was back down to my original xxx pounds. I stayed at that weight for most of the next twenty years. There were minor weight gains and losses, but for the most part my weight was stable and I didn't give it too much thought.

Nine years ago I got married. At the time, both my husband and I were working full time, and we ate out a lot. I gained about seven pounds, but I was really okay with that. Then, seven years ago, I developed a toothache. I went to the dentist. Her made a horrible mistake. I needed a root canal, but he was in a hurry to get to the office holiday party, so he decided to drill the tooth and put in a temporary filling. I was to come back the following week for a root canal. I never made it back for the root canal. The dentist sealed an infection into my tooth which, in turn went into my jaw. My jaw swelled. I couldn't open my mouth. I ended up having oral surgery to remove the infected tooth. For two months I was unable to open my mouth more than a tiny bit. My diet consisted of liquids and mushy things that could be sucked through a straw. This lasted almost two months. When I was finally up and around, I noticed that my clothes felt loose. I checked the scale, and sure enough, off came my post-marriage weight, plus some. I liked the feeling. And off I went on anther journey with my old enemy anorexia nervosa.

At the time, my husband was doing a job for his employer in north Las Vegas, and he came home only once a month. I know he was concerned, and he always asked if I was eating. By the time he returned home for good, it was too late. The anorexia had taken over yet again. I tried to fight it myself for the next couple of years. Finally, I couldn't stand to see the look of pain on my husband's face as he watched me slowly killing myself. I agreed to find treatment. There was a problem with my insurance, however. They would pay only for treatment in a hospital. All the eating disorder clinics in the area were outside a hospital setting.

We finally decided on outpatient treatment at a facility near our home in September 2014. I continued to go to the clinic for outpatient treatment until I made the decision to stop in January 2015. The treatment at the clinic was not what started me on my road to recovery, nor what kept me pushing on. What had actually started me on the road to recovery was my husband and the abandoned cat we had recently adopted. They deserved a wife and mommy who was whole and healthy. They loved me and I loved them, and ultimately I did not want to leave them behind.

I had heard from professionals that I needed to want to do this for myself for it to work, but I don't believe that to be true. I did it for my husband and my cat, and from that grew my desire to do this for myself. I wanted to be healthy again. I no longer wanted my life to be controlled by food, or lack of it. I gained back all the weight I had lost. I worked hard and my husband was proud of me.

I was proud of me.

I had a small setback when my cat passed away in October 2015, but I knew I could stop this before it got any worse. And I did. Dealing with an eating disorder, I believe, will always be a part of my life. It will always be lurking in the background, waiting for any of life's little setbacks to just give me a reason to give in to it. I will always have to fight it. But I believe that today I have the tools, and the love of myself and others, to keep me on the right path.

*

DENISE PURCELL
Denise is a 50-year-old living
with anorexia nervosa and bulimia

I was twelve years old, and remember being called the fat one when it came to family gatherings. I will never be pretty or thin enough; that's how my family judged people.

It started out small. I wouldn't eat breakfast and only picked at dinner. I managed to lose weight during a growth spurt and puberty; that was the last time I felt comfortable in my skin. I started getting noticed by boys, and my family stopped calling me fat. That was etched into my brain. In order to be loved or liked, you had to look perfect no matter what was going on in the inside. That became my motto in life.

I managed to maintain an acceptable weight up until I had my first daughter. I was young, just fifteen. The world was mine because I was skinny. And then I gained weight because I was pregnant. I gained it everywhere; it was the only time I felt safe enough to eat. I felt free. The baby was born, and again I was fat from the leftover weight. I began not eating again and doing exercises, and my weight went back down. This pattern continued with each pregnancy; I was in a sick cycle. Everything on the outside was fine, but my inner world was starving. I learned how to not feel hungry, and to hate food. My husband made me eat tuna and grapefruit, because he said I was disgusting, and looked better with my clothes on. I hated to be around people. I would hide. I bought diet pills, and went on every diet I could. I wanted to be so small, that maybe I would just disappear.

I weighed about xxx pounds when I noticed my reflection in the mirror, which I hated walking past. I could see my ribs. My collarbones protruded so much that it looked like a ditch. That scared me, because I had children to raise. I sought therapy. I realized the reasons why, and I know it's about control. I know all the right answers, and I did the opposite with my children. I made sure I didn't give them the same impression of how life works.

I was a prefect size two for over ten years. I knew the carb count of everything I ate. I snuck snacks at night and made myself throw up so it wouldn't change the scale. It was my own secret nightmare.

About two years ago I had my third back surgery. They inserted a screw through my nerve. I also had a radical hysterectomy that messed up my hormones, and took antidepressants that made me gain weight and lose mobility as I turned fifty. So now I weigh more than I ever have, even when I was pregnant. I want to hide, and don't go out much. I feel disgusting and judged and, although I know this is all in my head, it doesn't make it easier. I struggle with wanting to just be healthy.

*

HADDI TREBISOVSKY
Haddi is a 29-year-old living
with anorexia nervosa

There is something that I did once upon a time that was truly out of my comfort zone. I didn't realize it then, but this single decision would lead to the end of my seven-year-long battle with anorexia. This decision was terrifying. It was humiliating. It took everything in me not to give up. What was supposed to take one month ended up consuming six of my college months. I wept on the library's floor because of this decision. I covered my face with embarrassment when my boyfriend Jimmy, who's now my husband, tried comforting me. It was awful, yet I will still put my endorsement on this one because, when it was through, I had never been so free in my life.

Before I reveal this life-altering course of action, I need to explain a few things about myself. I have been blessed with two fabulous, thin, attractive parents who generously passed on their genes to me and my two gorgeous sisters. The three of us have never been overweight, and if beauty is measured based on society's expectations (which it should not be), we're doing all right. I'm not intending to brag. But you need to have this information to understand how tricky the devil can be with his lies, and how ridiculous my experience with the lies seemed to those around me.

It all started in ninth grade, when I was finally noticed by my male counterparts at school. It was exhilarating after having cried myself to sleep nearly every night in eighth grade because I did not have friends and nobody seemed to notice me. So at fourteen I started wearing clothes that were just a little tighter and a little shorter, and the reaction was pleasing. As the interaction between myself and these popular boys grew bolder, innocent teasing began to take place. I sat with them at lunch, and they began to comment on my lunch choices. Nothing was peculiar about what I was eating. But the teasing wasn't about what I was eating; it was about how much I was eating. Again, nothing peculiar about that. The boys thought it would be fun to tell me I was fat, and that I better slow down or skip this meal. Of course they were only flirting but after days, weeks and months of their flirting, I began to think that maybe I could stand to lose a few pounds. And I did. I lost ten pounds after deciding to skip lunches altogether.

Thus my eating disorder began. It was mild, and never landed me in the hospital. My parents were mostly unaware, but it consumed me. Everything I did made me conscious of how my body looked to others. Soon the consciousness of my body led to hatred of myself. I couldn't stand to look at myself, yet I couldn't be taken away from my mirror. It was an obsession that followed me everywhere. Even after attending what was essentially a year-long bible camp after high school, my self-image remained just barely above zero.

There are other parts of my story, particularly about suicide, depression, anxiety, and self-loathing, but for now I'll keep it focused on self-image. I tried heavier makeup, I tried coloring my hair, I tried different styles of clothing, I tried praying it away, I tried telling myself that I was beautiful in God's eyes. I tried telling myself that it's what's on the inside that counts. It all failed to open my eyes to any beauty that could be found inside me.

I was discouraged and disgusted with who I was. In my mind I was who I looked like, and what I looked like was not acceptable to me. No matter the number on the scale, it was never quite low enough and my stomach was never flat enough. By this point, I had been dating Jimmy for just a few months. We hadn't said we loved each other yet. This is when I made one very life-altering choice, and my boyfriend would suffer the consequences. Our church was initiating a month-long fast. Fasting from food has always been difficult and even unwise for me to participate in, because of the weight issue, but primarily because I am nearly guaranteed a migraine if I go too long without eating. I was contemplating how I could fast, and suddenly it hit me. It excited and terrified me simultaneously, but I knew what I had to do. I was going to fast from wearing makeup. Jimmy, the ever-supportive man that he is, was thrilled for me and this plan of action. He saw how his words did little to persuade me of the beauty he saw in me, so some outside help was more than welcome on his end.

So I washed my face that night and removed all my makeup. The first few days went all right—I knew this was what I was supposed to be doing, and the adrenaline overshadowed my fear. The fear of being exposed. The fear of being ugly. The fear of being plain. The fear of disenchanting my boyfriend. The fear of being worthless. But soon the adrenaline faded and reality set in. I was walking around in public without any makeup on, letting people see my raw, midwinter-pale face. Panic began to rise when I walked outside. Embarrassment at my condition kept me from making eye contact. I wanted to scream apologies to everyone who had to look at me throughout the day. I wanted everyone to know that this was only temporary—that they'd get the less ugly me soon enough. And then Jimmy had the guts to tell me I was beautiful.

I cringed, physically. I literally covered my face and did my best to plug my ears. He was wrong. He was cruel to lie to me in my weak position. He told me again. This time it was like a knife in my chest, just between the ribs, and it was twisting. The tears started burning, and I knew I was going to turn myself from ugly to hideous if I let the crying out. But I had no choice; he was still trying to convince me that he found me beautiful. It would have been okay if he told me I was beautiful on the inside but no, he meant the outside, and he was serious. Sobs came on full force and I wanted to scream.

If you've never had a lie exposed in yourself and had to fight it— let me tell you, those things do not go quietly. The enemy is sneaky, and he had been lying to me and I had been believing him for almost a decade. This lie had roots in me; it became part of me. Letting go of this lie was painful. It felt wrong to believe what Jimmy was telling me, what the Lord was trying to convey to me through my boyfriend's love and my peers' acceptance. You see, what happened was that people started talking to me more, they started complimenting me more. I was told over and over and over again how pretty I was without makeup. Unprompted. Without agenda. And slowly, over a month's time, the lie was being cut out of my heart.

By the time my month was over, I was a new creation. I looked in the mirror with gladness. I could accept my boyfriend's affections without guilt or shame. On the day my fast was finished, I decided I wasn't ready to put makeup back on. And for six months I didn't. Only after I went through this fast did I feel truly beautiful for the first time in my post-childhood life. And only after this fast did I recover from my eating disorder of seven years.

It has been over seven years since my makeup fast. I am honest when I say that self-image is no longer a problem for me. I do wear makeup, but I have learned how to have a healthy relationship with makeup, and I know that it does not define me. I've had two babies in this time, gaining over forty pounds with each pregnancy without batting an eye. I eat regular, healthy meals without worrying how it will affect my waistline. I am simply free from the bondage that food and self-image had imposed on me for so long.

As simple as it seems, it was a very difficult journey. I took away the enemy's tool to mess with me, and I haven't looked back since.

*

CHAPTER TWO

Realizing the Truth

> It is a great mystery that though the human heart longs for truth, in which alone it finds liberation and delight, the first reaction of human beings to truth is one of hostility and fear. -ANTHONY DE MELLO

Digesting the news of an eating disorder diagnosis can bring a flood of emotions. Guilt, shame, and even grief are common reactions. Further, our emotions vacillate like a rollercoaster, accepting one day and anger or denial the next. Or we might even pretend that we never received such a diagnosis. What was your reaction when you realized you had an eating disorder?

*

JUNE ALEXANDER
June is a 65-year-old living
beyond anorexia nervosa

I did not realize I had an eating disorder until some years after it had developed. I was a child, living on a family dairy farm in a rural area of southeastern Australia, when I developed anorexia nervosa.

My home did not have electricity connected, so there was no television, nor was there any literature that might have informed my parents about the onset of an eating disorder.

I was in my late teens and attending a larger school when I became more aware and realized that not everyone had the same inner struggles as me, and that I had an eating disorder. Shame and stigma, secrecy and isolation ruled my life. I had a secret life with the eating disorder, while trying to function like a "normal" person at school, with family and in relationships. Eventually, in my twenties, I would become suicidal. Not until my early thirties would a psychiatrist connect with the suppressed me, save my life and guide me to recovery over the next nineteen years.

Following is a description of the early days with my illness, an edited extract from my memoir, *A Girl Called Tim*, starting in 1962 when I was eleven years old.

I loved sleeping in my camp bed on the wooden veranda. Except for the bloody flies. As soon as the summer sun peeped over the hill and into our river valley, the dopey things woke up and started buzzing around my head. This particular January morning I tried to swat one that landed on my face. The sudden movement caused my narrow bed to wobble on its shaky legs, their rusty hinges creaking loudly. Oh well, the flies were a sign that it was time to get up anyway. I had big plans for the day.

School holidays were always fun on our family dairy farm, and the 1962 summer holidays held much promise. My days were full of helping my dad milk the cows, feeding the calves, shifting spray irrigation pipes, playing cricket with cousins and swimming in the river. At eleven I was a tomboy through and through, and proud of it. As I stirred in my bed, so did Topsy, my tortoiseshell cat. She burrowed under the covers and kept my feet warm during the chill of the night, but now she knew it was time to rise. I lay still for a moment and listened, beyond the buzz of the flies and Topsy's purr, to the gentle rumbling of rapids as the clear waters of the Mitchell River trundled over a stretch of rocks, five hundred meters down the hill from our farmhouse. The roosters were crowing, Rip the dog was barking, the cows were mooing and the milking machine engine was putt-putting away.

Our farm nestled at the head of the fertile Lindenow Valley, through which the river winded toward Bass Strait via Bairnsdale and the Gippsland Lakes, about thirty miles away. My parents had wed a few weeks after my mother's twenty-first birthday and lived in the same house as my grandparents. My sister Joy was born in 1948 and I followed on December 27, 1950. When I was five years old, my grandparents moved into a house in East Bairnsdale, twenty miles away. Joy and I sometimes stayed with them. This town life experience included a playground and milk bar in the same street, new friends with children across the road, and an occasional outing to the picture theater. Mostly I was desperately shy and sought shelter behind my sister.

My favorite grandmother, Grandma Alexander, died when I was ten. I was not taken to her funeral and I felt very lonely without her. She had patiently taught me, a left-hander, how to knit and crochet. I talked to Grandma in my prayers every night, telling her about my day, and how much I missed and loved her.

After my grandparents moved to Bairnsdale, their bedroom, that I had sometimes shared, became known as the "top bedroom" for guests. From the age of five to ten, when visitors required my bed as well, I slept on an inflatable rubber mattress on the floor of my parents' bedroom. By summer 1962, I was sleeping on the camp bed on the veranda. Visitors at this time of the year were mostly city cousins, and their parents, my Aunty Carlie and Uncle Roy. My cousins were allowed to sleep in, but I knew that when my mother came briskly out the back door, like now, I had two minutes in which to get up. That's how long she took to go out the back gate to the toilet to empty her chamber pot, rinse it under the garden tap and return it inside to its seclusion under her bed. I needed to jump out of bed before she came out the backdoor again, this time to sweep the concrete garden path. Otherwise, she would wave the broom to remind me that Dad was expecting his tea and toast. Besides, if I didn't get up right then, the flies would drive me crazy. I threw off the thin gray woolen blankets and swung out of bed, pulled on my shorts, T-shirt and gumboots, headed for the backdoor and yelled, "Mum, I'm ready to go to the dairy. Is Dad's tea and toast ready?" She loaded me up with a chipped enamel plate carrying several thick slices of high tin bread. The bread had been toasted on a homemade wire fork over embers in the firebox of our small, shiny black wood stove, and soaked with butter. An old saucepan lid was placed on top to keep the flies off. With this in one hand, I took the handle of the shining clean billy, half-filled with well-sugared black tea, in the other, and plodded in my roomy boots down the garden path, out the front gate and down the graveled track to the unpainted weatherboard dairy as fast as I could without slopping the tea or dropping the toast.

While I walked I thought about what the day would bring. My cousins and I had made plans the previous night for a maize cob fight in the stable after breakfast, followed by a swim in the river before lunch. My favorite swimmy hole was by the willows and windmill downstream from the rapids. There, depending on water flow, the river was about fifty meters wide and was bordered with a small sandy beach.

I took over milking our cows while Dad stood in our dairy's wash-up room and ate his toast, washing it down with a pannikin of tea poured from the billy. Our dairy herd of about forty-five cows was milked four at a time with machines powered by a diesel motor. By the age of eleven, I knew pretty much how everything worked as I'd been going to the dairy since I could walk. At first, my parents sold cream in cans that were collected by a lorry and taken to a butter factory in Bairnsdale. The leftover milk was fed to our pigs. Then we progressed to selling water-cooled milk. The milk, always deliciously warm, frothy and sweet fresh off the cows, was cooled as it ran over small stainless steel bars filled with water from an underground tank. After cooling it was stored in a big stainless steel vat until the milk tanker came, once or twice daily, to collect it. I managed to milk a few cows before Dad returned to the yard and then I fed the calves before carrying a billy of fresh milk up the hill for Mum to serve at breakfast. My lazy cousins were still in bed. Wondering where Mum was, I heard her call from up the hallway. I found her in her bedroom. Bother— what did she want? Mum closed her door. This seemed serious. "Tim, I have something to tell you." What had I done? "Did you notice anything when you got up this morning?" Notice anything? What? I hadn't made my bed but Mum usually made that for me while I was out helping Dad with the farm jobs. "No," I said. "Did you notice your pajamas, or look at your sheets?" she asked. What had I done? Had my cat made a mess? Couldn't have been me. "No," I said. "I found some blood," Mum said. "Blood? What blood?" Then Mum was talking. I could hear her but absorbed only snatches of what she said.

After talking about "periods" and "bleeding every month," she withdrew a small book from her dressing table drawer and told me to read it. The book's title was something like "Mothers and Daughters." I thought I'd read every book in the house long ago, but hadn't seen this one before. Then Mum pulled something from another of her dressing table drawers. It was a thin, circular elasticized belt with two dangly bits. From a bag in the depths of her wardrobe she pulled a white flannelette nappy. I watched, numbed and horrified. Spreading the nappy on the blue eiderdown of her freshly made bed, she folded it several times into a thick, narrow shape. Next, using two large safety pins from a little box on her dressing table, she attached the ends of the nappy to the two dangly bits. Mum held her work of art out toward me and said, "Wear this pad." I took it, speechless. My mother walked from the room, closing the door behind her. But not before pausing to add "And no swimming today, or tomorrow; not until you finish bleeding." I didn't want to hear any more. I felt disgusted. Me wear a nappy, a baby's thing?

Left alone, I slowly lowered my shorts and my pants. There was a little red patch. I took my pants off and pulled the bulky pad on. I felt a great need to escape that bedroom, and the house. I shoved the book under my camp bed pillow on the veranda, pulled on my gumboots and headed back to the dairy to help Dad wash the yards and clean up after the milking. As I walked down the track, kicking pebbles with my boots, I stopped. My mother's words hit hard, like a lightning strike. My world had changed forever. For a week every month I would have that bleeding—because I was a girl. I didn't want to be a girl; I wanted to be Tim. This is what Mum called me—well, when she was happy with me. When she was annoyed, she called me Toby. I'd wanted to be a boy for as long as I could remember. My boy cousins had shown me their "Willie" and I wanted one, too. My "Fanny" was a huge disappointment. At the age of six or seven I had lined up beside several boy cousins in the grassy calf paddock. Together we lowered our shorts and faced the timber wall of an old storage shed. We stood two meters out from the shed and our goal was to see who could "pee the highest" up the wall. "Ready, set, go!" The boy's wee reached almost as high as the shed roof. I leaned back and pushed as hard as I could but mine didn't go beyond the toe of my gumboots. Most of the warm yellow liquid fell directly south into my boots, soaking my socks and making my feet squelch and smell. Not having a Willie was frustrating but to learn that my Fanny would bleed once a month was devastating. I shook myself and trudged on to the dairy. I was sure I was as handy as a boy in all other ways. I preferred farm work to house jobs. Besides feeding the calves twice a day and helping with the cows, I set rabbit traps, drove the tractor and helped to shift the irrigation pipes.

Would Dad notice I was different? He said nothing as I entered the dairy to sweep and hose the yards and help put water through the pipes to clean the machines now the last cow had been milked. But that stupid *nappy was chaffing my inner legs. I hoped it wasn't bulging through my shorts. By now it was nine o'clock. I walked back up the hill for breakfast. My sleepy cousins were starting to appear. They said nothing. Just as well they didn't know about this sudden complication in my life. They would laugh if they knew I was wearing a nappy. After breakfast, in the stable downhill from the house, we drew an imaginary battle line and prepared for the maize cob fight. We gathered old, shelled cobs off the dusty dirt floor for ammunition, hid among the bales of hay, old machinery and hessian bags brimming with full cobs, and the war started. Mum growled if we threw full cobs, as they were food for the chooks, but in the heat of battle we threw them anyway. That day we decided the Allies were invading Germany. The cobs, especially if unshelled, hurt if they struck bare skin, and that was our aim. We had to draw blood on the enemy, usually on their face or arms, to claim victory.*

Waging war helped me to momentarily forget my other bloody problem, but I had to mumble, "Mum wants me to do a job in the house," when my cousins asked why I wasn't going for a swim. "Chicken," they said. The next few days seemed like years. And then I was free to go swimming again, between helping Dad with the cows and shifting the irrigation pipes on our twenty-four hectares of river flats.

My happiness was short-lived. In the first week of February, I pedaled my bike out of the valley to attend the local state school, Woodglen Primary, Number 3352, two and a half miles away. Surrounded by farmland and flanked on three sides by tall pine trees, the school comprised one classroom. We had a porch to hang our bags, and the little children listened to "Kindergarten of the Air." We had a tiny storeroom for our sports equipment. I was in grade six, my final year of primary school. One of my cousins was the teacher, and had been since grade four. He had grown up in Melbourne but I knew him well as, along with many other cousins and family friends, he often stayed at our house. It was a favorite place for everyone to visit.

There were five girls and three boys in grade six, the biggest in the school, which had a total enrollment of twenty-four children. Most of our parents were dairy farmers. Some, like my parents, owned their property; others, including a Dutch family with thirteen children, share farmed on a larger property. I enjoyed learning but something about my teacher cousin made me uneasy. Every morning we stood beside our wooden desks. He said, "Good morning boys and girls." We would chorus, "Good morning," and his name, before sitting down to work. Except I refused to say his name. He was my cousin after all, and only twelve years older. He wouldn't let me call him by his first name at school, so I called him nothing. My mother and sister Joy called me stubborn and pigheaded. I didn't care. There was something about this cousin that had me on edge, and it was not just his name.

When he first came to our school I was nine. Every Monday morning, we lined up by the weatherboard shelter shed for a flag-raising ceremony and sang "God Save the Queen." While standing at attention with my hand over my heart one morning several weeks into Term One, I glanced along the line and my heart went thump as I realized I was the only girl with breasts. When I ran, my breasts bounced up and down and hurt. If I held them, they didn't hurt. But I couldn't do that when playing with the boys or within sight of the teacher.

In March, the teacher announced that the school doctor, who visited our school each three or four years, would come in June. He gave us forms for our parents to fill in and sign. I gave my form to Mum, saying I didn't want to see the doctor but she said, "Don't be silly, you have nothing to worry about, Tim. It will be over in a flash, you'll see."

Her words provided no comfort. I would have to undress to my panties and singlet. Maybe I would have to take off my singlet as well. I'd be in the classroom, which had large multi-paned windows on two sides, and no curtains. For a reason I could not explain, I was extremely fearful of my teacher cousin seeing me undressed. My sister, Joy, brushed my concerns aside. Our cousin hadn't been her teacher as she started high school at Bairnsdale, the year he came to Woodglen, three years ago now. We shared the same bedroom and our cousin gave her the creeps too, but when I said I didn't want to see the doctor, she said, "All the other girls will be undressing; you won't be the only one." But I would be the only one with sissy breasts. This was definitely something I couldn't talk to Dad about. I had nobody else to turn to.

The doctor's visit was only three months away and my breasts were growing bigger. Soon I would need to wear a bra. Sitting on the grassy school ground in the shade of the pine trees during playtime one Friday afternoon, there seemed no way to avoid this doctor's visit. Suddenly, however, I knew what to do. It was as though my brain was zapped from outer space. Ping! I was unaware that anorexia nervosa was developing and beginning to manipulate my mind. I only knew I felt less anxious. Classmates were calling me to come and play; they could not see my special new thought "friend."

That very afternoon, when classes resumed, a serendipitous health lesson provided encouragement. With other pupils I sat cross-legged on a carpet square with my health booklet to listen to the voice booming from our big wireless. It described a new word: c-a-l-o-r-i-e. A day earlier the word would have held no interest but now my mind clung to it like a magnet. The lesson was about food values and burning energy. My booklet listed the calorie content of several foods and the number of calories absorbed in thirty minutes of walking, swimming, running and bike riding. My mind recorded the entire lesson word for word and I immediately began to eat less and exercise more. When tempted to eat, I pushed my hunger pangs aside. The hungrier I was, the better I felt. If feeling weak, I brushed my teeth, which helped me think I had eaten a meal, though I'd eaten nothing.

I had no idea of my weight. The only scales I had seen were those belonging to the school doctor, or those with a penny slot outside chemist *shops in Bairnsdale's Main Street. I went to town three or four times a year and was too shy to weigh myself in view of passers-by. All I knew was that I wanted to lose my breasts before the school doctor's visit.*

Until now, I had been pleased when my clothes became tight, because this showed I was growing, and I wanted to be tall and strong, like Dad. But now I didn't want to grow. I could not be like my dad, and didn't want to be a girl, either. I continued to feed the calves before riding my bike to school, but did my jobs faster so I could work out on the playground equipment before lessons started. I swung across the monkey bars and, like a monkey after a coconut, shinned up the pole. I reached for the clouds on the swing, did chin-ups, climbed the ladder, zipped down the slide, and turned myself inside out on the jungle gym. I worked out again at playtime and lunchtime, counting and always increasing the number of turns on each piece of equipment.

At home I chopped more wood, looked after the chooks and fetched the cows for milking, running from job to job. Mum and Dad thought I was wonderful. Mum was calling me "Tim" all the time, I was so helpful, but my parents did not know that an illness was driving me to do more and more physical activity each day, and to eat less food every day. Exercise was easy but eating less was more complicated as Mum was in charge of the kitchen. Breakfast was straightforward. Mum was usually helping Dad in the dairy when I was in the house changing out of my cow yard gear into my school clothes. She'd leave the table set with Weet-Bix on a plate or porridge keeping warm in the saucepan on the side of the stove, thick slices of bread on a plate to toast and tea in the pot. Joy would have left an hour earlier to catch the bus to high school; and any visitors would be still in bed. The cats loved the porridge and Weet-Bix. Besides Topsy, we had about twelve cats. Some were part feral, having been dumped by uncaring owners in the bush land adjacent to our property. Timid, they lived in the stable and haystack where they caught mice; some bravely hung around the back door of the house in the mornings and evenings, hoping for a dish of stale milk, or scraps from the kitchen.

They purred as I fed them my cereal, telling them to eat it up before Mum returned from the dairy. Next I took a thick slice of high tin loaf outside, through the back gate, throwing chunks to the chooks, who snapped the bread up in their beaks and dashed about, clucking madly and throwing their heads back as they gulped their treat down. Then I ran back inside, cut a paper-thin slice of bread to toast on the open fire, spread some Vegemite and washed it down with a cup of black, sugarless tea. From the age of five I'd been drinking tea from a favorite cup that Mum half-filled with milk, and sweetened with several teaspoons of white sugar. Not anymore. Every day I found new ways to reduce my calorie intake. Lunch on school days was easy, too. Mum cut two big rounds of sandwiches, wrapping them in waxed paper and placing them in my blue lunch tin, the lid kept on with an old Vacola ring. I asked for only one round but she wouldn't listen and when I came home from school with one sandwich untouched, she was upset. "You need two rounds, you're a growing girl and besides, this is wasteful," Mum scolded. I thought of another solution. The next day I took an empty tin home. "That's better," Mum said. Some schoolchildren came from poor families who sometimes had no bread to make lunch, so I offered my sandwiches to these children. I gave them the cheese, jam, meat and peanut butter sandwiches, keeping a Vegemite, fish paste or tomato one for myself. My classmates also enjoyed my play snacks of lamingtons, jam drops, Madeira cake, chocolate slice and Anzac biscuits. I smiled as they ate while I went hungry; I enjoyed watching them eat.

The evening meal was the one daily meal shared by my family. Mum served the food on our plates and set them on the oval-shaped, oak dining table that stood in the middle of our kitchen. I dreaded casseroles, stews and gravy. Desserts were particularly messy. I became resourceful and devious. By sitting down first, when Mum's back was turned at the sink and others were combing their hair before coming to the table, I had time to move food from my plate to the next plate, which belonged to whoever was visiting. This pleased me. I liked to watch people eat. If I didn't particularly like them, I liked to think that they were getting fatter and fatter. If Mum left the kitchen for a moment, I risked reaching across the table and placing my meat on Dad's plate. Sometimes I gave his plate a roast potato as well. These were his favorite foods, and Dad was my favorite person in all the world. When everyone was seated and busy eating or talking, I grabbed fistfuls of food left on my plate, whipped it under the tablecloth and slid it in my pockets. This was why I didn't like sloppy foods like mashed potato and meat covered in gravy. I ate a small amount of cabbage or carrot and pretend it was a lot, chewing it over and over, finishing my meal at the same time as everyone else.

Main courses were a trial but desserts were worse. They were sticky or soft and hopeless for slipping in pockets. Mum made chocolate sauce puddings, apple crumbles, apple puddings, golden syrup dumplings, jam tarts, sago puddings and custards, usually served with stewed or preserved fruit. Made with full-cream milk and butter, the desserts also contained sugar, available by the cupful from a big hessian bag in our pantry. My heart sank when Mum insisted on pouring custard sauce or cream over the top of a steamed pudding. About the only dessert I could slip safely in my pocket was cinnamon apple cake, and even that was messy. I tried to tell Mum, "I am full. I don't want dessert, thank you." But she would say, "What's wrong with you? I thought you wanted to be tall and strong like your Dad." Nothing but a cleaned-up plate satisfied my mother. She would remind me how as a child she had "bread and dripping through the week and bread and jam on Sunday" and for good measure would add, "Think about those poor starving children in India, be grateful and eat up." I couldn't see how the eating of my dessert would ease the plight of children in India. I wanted to lose my breasts. I couldn't tell her that, so I waited for everyone to leave the table and for Mum to leave the kitchen, even for a moment. Then I'd jump up and toss the food off my plate into the scrap bowl and run it outside in the dark to Rip the dog, whose turn it was for a meal at the end of the day. Rip developed a real sweet tooth.

Summer passed into autumn, and autumn was nearing winter. My periods were on time every month. At school, I remained the only girl with breasts but they were shrinking and I hid them by wearing more clothing as the weather turned cooler. However, Mum was starting to question my behavior. On weekends, I liked to disappear into the bushland adjacent to our property, my thoughts as my companion. My mother and sister called me "stuck-up" and "rude" when I didn't want to join them in visiting our neighbors, who put the kettle on for a cuppa, whatever the time of day, and served sugar-laden cakes and biscuits. I had friends on neighboring farms but preferred to be alone or doing outdoor jobs. Luckily Mum liked me to help Dad and I was with him every possible moment. She worked hard, helping on the farm when I was at school and she kept our house spotless and large cottage garden beautiful.

Some local families had electric power, but it hadn't entered our valley yet, so Mum did her housework manually: polishing the linoleum floors on her hands and knees, beating her cake mixtures with a wooden spatula, and washing our clothes in a wood-fired copper. She prodded the clothes with a broken ax handle before heaving them into a concrete trough to rinse in cold water, and wrung them by hand before pegging them on the outside line. The steel-bladed Southern Cross windmill by the river provided our water supply, pumping water to a tank one hundred meters uphill from the house to gain sufficient pressure. Careful usage was essential because otherwise, when wind didn't blow, the tank ran dry. One night, lost in thought over how to avoid the shepherd's pie that Mum was baking for tea, I forgot to turn off the tap into the calves' trough. Next morning, Dad gently asked, "Did you forget to do something last night?" The tank had run dry. I hung my head. I would not forget again.

The following week the doctor came to school. My chest was almost flat. As far as I could tell, my teacher cousin stayed out of sight. Nobody laughed as I lined up with the other girls in panties and singlets, the doctor chatted, probed and listened to each of us in turn before passing us on to the nurse who weighed us. At xxx pounds, neither the doctor nor nurse noted a weight loss because they hadn't seen me for four years. My report was good on every count. While dressing I looked sideways and was pleased to notice other Grade Six girls were growing breasts too. I had worked hard for three months, preparing for the doctor's visit. Now it was over. That afternoon, pushing my bike through the school gate to pedal home, I felt relieved I wouldn't risk making Mum cross at mealtime anymore. But the eating disorder was going nowhere fast.

*

OLIVIA ANTHONY
Olivia is a 44-year-old living
with anorexia nervosa and bulimia

I vividly remember the exact moment I realized that I had bulimia. I was relieved and also felt real. Like, because I had bulimia, I mattered enough to get help. My history started out with anorexia, but I just figured I was healthier and had better self-control than others. Two years prior, my roommate made an appointment for both of us with a campus minister because she saw that we were anorexic and needed help. I left the waiting room before the minister called us back. I just didn't see that I had a problem. But, after I slipped into bulimia, I felt like a fraud and a loser. I felt like a fraud because with the amount of food I was eating, I should have been huge. But I was cheating at life and purging it all up. I was out of control. I felt awful physically and emotionally. So after purging on that cold Minnesota day, I went for a walk and did the math in my head. I remembered reading a book about eating disorders that said in order to be considered bulimic, you had to purge twice a week for three months.

I was purging xxx times a day for that long. I said out loud, "I'm bulimic!" I was relieved. I had a legitimate illness and could get help. I was so lonely and felt so out of control. I was desperately hopeful that someone could help get me out of the mental hell I was in.

*

CHRISTINE BASTONE
Christine is a 49-year-old living
with binge eating disorder

I hadn't really thought of myself as having an eating disorder until very recently. Oh, I knew I had a problem with food. I even believed I was addicted to food. But I don't have anorexia or bulimia that I typically think of as an eating disorder. I binge, sure, but I don't purge. So thinking of myself as someone with an eating disorder is very new for me.

*

LYNDA CHELDELIN FELL
Lynda is a 50-year-old living
with binge eating disorder

I didn't realize I had an eating disorder until I was forty years old. I had known for a long time that I had virtually no control over food, especially sweets. But like a lot of Americans, I just thought of myself as fat, not as having an eating disorder. I had gained and lost a hundred pounds more than once. But when I realized that all it took was one nibble to trigger a hundred-pound binge, deep down I knew I had something more than obesity.

The truth is that I felt too ashamed to say anything to my doctor, or ask for help of any kind. Who talks about binge eating? Nobody I knew. Anorexia and bulimia were eating disorders but, from what I could tell, society didn't view bingeing as anything other than gluttonous. Compassion and pity were readily offered to the anorexic individual. After the singer Karen Carpenter died, it was identified as a truly dangerous disease that threatened one's life. But disgust was the only reaction offered an obese person. After all, nobody twisted our arm to eat that Big Mac (or two). So my initial reaction at realizing I had a problem, a true eating disorder, was shame and hopelessness.

*

JUSTINE HILDEN
Justine is a 27-year-old living
with binge eating disorder

I gained a significant amount of weight during my freshman year of college, but I was able to lose it over the summer before my sophomore year. After that I just started eating, and in turn gaining weight. I continued to hit weights that I had never seen before. It never once crossed my mind that I had an eating disorder. I thought that maybe there was something wrong with my thyroid, or something else, I'm not even sure what.

I spent time online searching and checking out all kinds of things. I saw my doctor and after all my blood work came back normal, she talked to me about the depression and anxiety I had been diagnosed with in my freshman year. She started talking about my eating habits. She mentioned The Emily Program, but I kind of blew it off. I got home and began research. I always thought of eating disorders as anorexia and bulimia. I never thought there was an eating disorder for people who ate a lot and who gained weight like I did. It's become more common and more talked about now, but even eight years ago or so, I wasn't familiar with the terms binge eating disorder or compulsive overeating. After further internet searching, I knew that's what I was dealing with.

I felt relief in being able to identify it. But at the same time I felt ashamed, embarrassed, scared, overwhelmed, angry, frustrated, and every other emotion in between. I couldn't believe I had a problem. I was always normal. I truly thought that this would never happen to me, but it did. I can still visualize showing my mom a description of my eating disorder and telling her, "This is exactly what I'm dealing with." I then began my first time at The Emily Program.

*

LYDIA KENYON
Lydia is a 22-year-old living
with anorexia nervosa

I think that after a certain point I knew I had an issue with eating, and suspected it could be an eating disorder. I wasn't sure, though, because I was home-schooled and uneducated about mental illness and eating disorders. My mom became very concerned and began making phone calls, which was when she confirmed our fears: I had anorexia.

*

REBEKKAH KOONS
Rebekkah is a 29-year-old living with an
eating disorder not otherwise specified

I first realized I had an eating disorder when my best friend told me I was getting too skinny. Instead of being concerned, I was actually happy and satisfied with that comment. It felt like a trophy.

*

MONICA MIRKES
Monica is a 58-year-old living
with binge eating disorder

Denial. Anger. Hopelessness. I knew I was headed in the wrong direction with my weight, but didn't want to admit it. I hated that I couldn't control what I ate. I would justify the banana splits, snowballs and candy bars. I felt that my life was spiraling down the drain and I wasn't even going to try to stop myself. Complete indifference. It's horrible to admit even now. I would just tell myself, "Oh, well. This is how it's going to be. I deserve it for not being able to take control of my actions."

*

RUTH PAPALAS
Ruth is a 58-year-old living
with binge eating disorder

I didn't realize I had a disorder. I thought I was just fat. So I guess I would say I was in denial. Who wants to admit any kind of disorder? Especially one where all you have to do is not overeat. I was very upset when the singer Karen Carpenter died from anorexia. It seemed that all she would have had to do was hang out with me, eat what I ate, and she would still be singing her beautiful songs. I didn't understand or realize at the time that there was such a thing as anorexia or anything that would constitute an eating disorder. I never gave a thought to an eating disorder affecting me. I kept gaining weight, thinking that someday it would just fall off.

*

DEBBIE PFIFFNER
Debbie is a 56-year-old living
with anorexia nervosa

My eating disorder began in 1977 at the age of seventeen. At that time, very little was known about eating disorders. Very few people even knew there was such a disease. I found out I had an eating disorder when I read an article about anorexia nervosa in *Reader's Digest*, and the article described me. There was a girl in my class at school who had a sister who had anorexia. She tried to get me to talk to her sister on many occasions. I had mixed feelings when I realized that I did indeed have an eating disorder. A part of me was scared. I knew I could die from this disease. There were nights when I didn't want to fall asleep because I didn't know if I would wake up the next morning. Part of me was also validated every time I was told I was too thin. That was such a compliment. What could be better than being too thin? Coming from a family where I never felt wanted, it was nice to finally get attention, even if that attention came from my parents arguing over me, or with me, begging or screaming at me to eat.

My family, my friends, even the doctors didn't understand why I refused to eat. That gave me a sense of being a little special. People treated me differently—they sometimes walked on eggshells around me so as not to upset me and make me worse. That gave me a type of power I had never had. I did not purposefully prolong my disease in any way just for attention or power—I knew I was seriously in trouble and I knew I did not want to die. It was a mixed bag of feelings that even I did not quite know how to handle.

When my eating disorder reared again twenty years later, I think my biggest emotion was shame. Shame that I had allowed something that I thought was under control to come back, and shame that I was hurting my husband so badly. He tried so desperately to understand and be supportive.

I will admit that over the course of my life, and through both bouts with anorexia, I have felt anger at everyone. I thought, why can't you just leave me alone? But I also know that it was never an option for anyone who cared about me to just leave me alone.

*

DENISE PURCELL
Denise is a 50-year-old living
with anorexia and bulimia

When I first realized I had an eating disorder I felt ashamed. I felt like it was a secret that no one could know or understand. This was before eating disorders were ever talked about. I knew it was wrong but it didn't matter, because I had to make myself perfect in order to be accepted and loved by my family and friends and the world. No matter where you are, it's everywhere, including magazines and television all talking about facelifts and diets, and who wouldn't want to look like a model? Everyone looks at models. Somehow I had to raise myself to achieve those standards, no matter what. As long as I received compliments, it continued. My health didn't matter, I didn't matter. My emotions and thought processes were so out of whack that I felt I had no control over anything in my life. At least with not eating or overeating I called the shots.

*

HADDI TREBISOVSKY
Haddi is a 29-year-old living
with anorexia nervosa

It's hard for me to recall a particular moment when I first became aware that skipping meals and holding myself back from eating a whole portion of food was a disordered eating pattern. I do remember, though, feeling a sense of gratification and satisfaction that finally something was wrong with me. Back in middle and high school, in the early stages of my anorexia, I was a far more emotionally driven girl than I am now. Not just moody, but I felt things much more deeply than my peers did. I could be distraught over a friend's troubles to the point where I'd lose sleep and it would be all I could think of, even though it didn't directly affect me. I had depressive and anxious tendencies that often led to self-hatred. So when I realized that what I was doing was unhealthy and wrong, I felt pleased that I was punishing and disciplining myself in the way I thought I needed to. I also felt as though I had an upper hand when friends and peers commented on their weight versus mine, and I was glad to have the (perceived) self-control that I did in order to skip meals. I also fully accepted that this would need to be how I lived from then on if I wanted to maintain a thin form for the rest of my life, so I was always proud if I could push through a meal or snack, even if it meant that a headache followed.

*

After all these years, I am still involved in the process of self-discovery. It's better to explore life and make mistakes than to play it safe.
SOPHIA LOREN

*

CHAPTER THREE

The Familial Link

My family is my strength and my weakness.
-AISHWARYA RAI BACHCHAN

Once upon a time, eating disorders were often attributed to overly controlling parents. Within the last few years research has uncovered other predispositions, opening the door to the possibility of familial links. Do other family members struggle with an eating disorder?

*

JUNE ALEXANDER
June is a 65-year-old living
beyond anorexia nervosa

Upon reflection, I can see that my mother suffered anxiety, and her eating behaviors were not a good role model for me. For instance, she would eat from a bread-and-butter plate, or a saucer, rather than a normal dinner plate. She was always on the move, and this seems to have been her way of coping with her anxiety. She was always doing things for others, but refused to talk to me about my eating disorder. Toward the end of her life, when I was writing my memoir, she told me she had burned all photographs taken of me during my childhood and early adolescence when anorexia was severe, because she hated to look at them. When I was a child, she had the effect of making me feel guilty if I sat down to read a book. She would say, "You should be outside helping your father on the farm; you know he is so tired," and this had an effect that lasted into my adulthood. I would feel guilty if I sat down to read, or just be. My sister would binge eat. A cousin developed anorexia. My childhood friends did not develop an eating disorder. I was the only one in my peer group with this illness.

*

OLIVIA ANTHONY
Olivia is a 44-year-old living
with anorexia nervosa and bulimia

No one else in my family has been diagnosed with an eating disorder. In 2001 my parents and I gave our blood samples for a genetic study about eating disorders. We had questionnaires to fill out as well. They didn't ever tell us the test results, but I'm convinced that there is a genetic component. There has to be. I'm sure my sister has orthorexia. She exercises to an extreme, and is obsessed about food and weight. She denies she has a problem, but it's pretty clear that she does. My paternal grandma is really overweight. She was always on a diet, talked about weight, and regularly asked me what size I was. I hated that! She was obsessed with food and weight. My mom used to be an emotional eater, and got pretty heavy. She doesn't struggle with it now, but she sure did when she was with my dad. He was a controlling person. I remember him taking food from my mom because he didn't think she should have it. While in high school I easily hid ED. My dad is naturally scrawny and all of us kids were also thin. No one knew what I was up to, because I had always been naturally under-weight. In college, my roommate confided in me that she had anorexia and bulimia in her past. Well, from the beginning it was obvious that she still struggled. We both ended up eating the same exact things. We used to count calories together and compete with each other. I have had a few friends over the years who confided that they used to be anorexic or bulimic. I've only had a couple of friends who were actively eating disordered at the same time as me.

*

CHRISTINE BASTONE
Christine is a 49-year-old living
with binge eating disorder

I don't believe any members of my family struggle with an eating disorder. I assume that between my offline and online friends, a few of them do, although I have no idea which ones.

*

LYNDA CHELDELIN FELL
Lynda is a 50-year-old living
with binge eating disorder

Obesity runs in my family, as do addiction and depression. Food is used for comfort by most of my siblings, though we rarely acknowledge it. Only one of my four children, our youngest son, inherited binge eating and lack of satiety. He was obese until he was fifteen, and then shed nearly a hundred pounds and has since kept it off. I had never heard about anorexia until the singer Karen Carpenter died. I couldn't believe somebody died of self-induced starvation! What a strange disease she had. As a binge eater, it feels like my end of the spectrum is largely ignored. I've since become more vocal about being a food addict, and have had some open conversations with our son so he doesn't feel as alone as I did. I've also been more vocal about my binge eating within the extended family. It is important to give voice to the struggle so future generations don't inherit the same stigma.

*

JUSTINE HILDEN
Justine is a 27-year-old living
with binge eating disorder

In high school, I had friends who struggled with anorexia and bulimia. I thought they were crazy. I couldn't wrap my head around how someone could have such a weird and dysfunctional relationship with food. I remember confronting them about it. It doesn't run in my family. I never knew a family member to be diagnosed with an eating disorder. I do have an extensive family history of depression, anxiety, alcoholism, and drug addiction. Even though they say addiction is different, and I believe it is, there are definitely some similarities. I used to hang out with a woman whom I had met in my intensive outpatient program. It helped to be around women who were like me, struggled with food like me, and had experiences similar to mine. We knew so much about each other, things that no one else knew because we went through treatment together. As I have gone farther in my recovery process, I have had to distance myself from many of them, because our paths were going in different directions. They will always have a special place in my heart, but it's best for me to go my separate way while I try to get my life back.

*

LYDIA KENYON
Lydia is a 22-year-old living
with anorexia nervosa

Growing up, I knew no one who had an eating disorder. No one in my family had an eating disorder that I know of. Now that I am in the recovery process, I do know a few women who have eating disorders, and hearing their stories has been an experience that makes me feel understood and supported.

*

REBEKKAH KOONS
Rebekkah is a 29-year-old living with
an eating disorder not otherwise specified

My cousin opened up to me about her struggles with bulimia, but my family is very closed to talking about feelings. Even though they knew, no one ever said it out loud or confronted me. It was the same with my friends. They didn't say anything, probably because they didn't understand, which is no one's fault. My online ED friends were all I needed at the time anyway.

*

MONICA MIRKES
Monica is a 58-year-old living
with binge eating disorder

I remember as a teenager my mother getting and taking weight-loss pills and Valium. There was a pill for everything. I used to tell her that thanks to her generation's abuse, my generation had to work it off and deal with life. I have friends in the same boat, trying to lose weight, willing to try anything that even hints of weight-loss benefits. I had one friend who talked about tapeworms!

*

RUTH PAPALAS
Ruth is a 58-year-old living
with binge eating disorder

Several of my friends and family members struggle with their weight, but I do not believe that they have a disorder. Even if they did, they would not admit it. They would say that they just enjoy eating and if they wanted to lose weight they could just go on a diet.

*

DEBBIE PFIFFNER
Debbie is a 56-year-old living
with anorexia nervosa

As far as I know, no one in my immediate or extended family has ever had an eating disorder. I knew one girl in my high school who had anorexia, but I never spoke to her about it until after we were both well into recovery. Then we shared our thoughts and feelings. Finally I had someone to talk with who understood what I was going through, and all the feelings that came along with the disease itself, and with recovery. Prior to that, I was very alone. Eventually we lost touch with each other. At the time when my eating disorder was at its worst, I had no one who understood what I was going through, and I know there were people in my life who thought I was just stubborn, that I enjoyed the attention and was doing this because it's what I wanted to do. No one understood the anxiety that accompanies an eating disorder; how eating just a morsel of food would send my anxiety to extremes. That this was something I couldn't control, not something I chose to do.

Later in my life I had a very good friend who suffered from anorexia and bulimia throughout her life. We constantly checked on each other. We asked each other things like: Have you been eating? Did you lose weight? We freely discussed our eating disorders with each other, knowing we were in the same boat. We could also go to each other if we felt we were heading for trouble. She has since passed away from cancer, and when my eating disorder flared up again, I truly missed having her to help me through. There is a friend whom I see periodically. One day we were having a conversation and I said to her, "It's probably obvious since I'm wearing shorts and a tank top, but I have an eating disorder." She smiled at me and said, "Debbie, I've known all along." I asked her how she knew, and her response was, "It takes one to know one." Although I don't see her very often, whenever I do I get excited to tell her that I've gained weight and what progress I'm making. She listens, understands, and makes me feel not alone.

*

DENISE PURCELL
Denise is a 50-year-old living
with anorexia nervosa and bulimia

I don't think my family or friends knew or cared about eating disorders; they were never concerned or showed any interest unless it was to call out someone who was overweight in their eyes. My extended family, my aunts, always commented on weight. I think all women had that same way of thinking. Overweight was gross and no one would love you. I believe it was another dirty secret kept by many women.

*

HADDI TREBISOVSKY
Haddi is a 29-year-old living
with anorexia nervosa

As far as I know, no one in my family struggles or struggled with an eating disorder. I did not begin my ED knowing anyone else with an ED, but later on one of my friends developed anorexia.

*

CHAPTER FOUR

Hiding the Secrets

We have much to learn by studying nature and taking the time to tease out its secrets. - DAVID SUZUKI

Eating disorders encompass more than just food. An estimated sixty percent of women eat in secret because of shame and other negative emotions. While we know that the thought patterns make no logical sense, we are powerless to stop. And thus a pattern of secrets begins. What extremes have you gone to in order to hide your eating disorder?

*

JUNE ALEXANDER
June is a 65-year-old living
beyond anorexia nervosa

My memoir, *A Girl Called Tim*, reveals the extent and inherent danger to health and relationships, in seeking to appease the eating disorder's incessant demands and hide its relationship with me.

I lived in a rural social environment in the 1960s and 1970s, when mental illness was considered a weakness. Attempts to explain my inner struggles were invalidated with comments like "Pull up your socks," "You think about yourself too much," and "Why can't you be like other girls in the district?" Eventually I suppressed my struggles within, which pleased my eating disorder immensely, and hastened complete disintegration of my authentic self from my body. Sometimes, my silent food fight manifested outwardly. This memoir excerpt is from 1971, when I was twenty.

Gee, I never know what the next day will bring —I washed my hair in the bath tonight, and as I was getting out, I started to get dizzy and my heart went bang, bang. I got out and opened the door, sat on the chair and then I blacked out and I don't remember what happened next. Must have fallen on the floor with a bang, 'cos Mum came running. Must have given her a bad fright. She ran up the passage and shouted for Dad, and then I came round. I lay on my bed and oh, I now have a very empty tummy. Mum wants me to go to the doctor, but I feel okay now, and Dad says that's the main thing. Don't think I'll wash my hair in the bath again... Mum says I need rest and food?! I said I will be early to bed.

I was eating enough food, but was stuffing myself one day and starving myself the next. I tried, but could not eat three meals a day like "normal" people. I constantly felt that something wasn't right, but if I weighed xxx kg, everything will be right. I didn't know such thoughts were not normal or that my incessant battle to ease anxiety by counting calories was a sign of illness. Food consumed ninety-five percent of my think time.

April 10, 1971, my wedding day. 11:15 a.m. Hairdressers. I was up soon after 7 a.m. I had a bath and washed my hair and then I had a blackout. I have a big headache from when I hit the floor. I lay on Mum's bed until I recovered—my stomach lost its contents! I weighed just xxx! I had trouble remembering what day it was. Had two mugs of soup for breaky—not eating anything more until the reception. I'm going to eat each of the four courses!

The eating disorder and chaos accompanied me into my marriage. The morning of Friday, June 18, started badly.

George and I slept in until 6.45 a.m., and arose to find our hot and cold water taps frozen. Most annoying! George went to milk the cows and all I could do before leaving for work was vacuum the floors and make the bed. While doing so I ate ten fruit scones to quell my nagging emptiness. I had been married ten weeks and already my happiness was being sabotaged.

Driving to work along the Omeo Highway with my mind sluggish and my stomach stuffed with scones, I was ascending a long slope known as the Sandhill when I pulled out to overtake a loaded cattle truck. The truck seemed to blow brown exhaust smoke across my windscreen and, unable to see, I started to return to the left side of the road, in case there was oncoming traffic. At the same time, I reached for the wiper switch on the left of my steering wheel to improve vision, but before I could, I was knocked unconscious. Then I felt like Alice in Wonderland, being drawn up out of a deep, dark burrow. I slowly opened and raised my eyes and began taking in my surroundings. Blood was trickling down my pale gray woolen coat, the dashboard was covered in shattered glass, and I was slumped on the passenger side of the front seat.

This was a bad dream, but as my eyes gained focus, reality dawned: I'd driven into the back of a big log truck, now stopped in front of my car. Three huge logs on it. I was sandwiched between the cattle truck, which had stopped behind me, and the log truck. The police ran checks on the cattle truck, but found nothing amiss. They were so impressed with my survival that they placed a photo of my car in their station window. Seatbelt legislation was about to be introduced in Victoria and a policeman said, "If you had been restrained by a belt, the big log that went through the windscreen over your steering wheel might have decapitated you." Privately, I believed that my scone binge may have clouded my driving judgment, but I dare not mention it. People would think I was silly. The facts were that I hadn't seen the log truck and had been transported "to the other side" where peace reigned, and drawn back again. Everyone agreed I was lucky to be alive.

Three years later, in 1974, the eating disorder was affecting not only my health and my relationship with my husband, but also my children. With two little boys to keep me occupied, everything was rosy in my world except for the sleepless nights, the problem of George being dissatisfied with his job, and my inner void. Within a few weeks of (second son) Rohan's birth, my bingeing caused upsets in my breast milk and consequently upsets in Rohan, who vomited three times in one night. This regular occurrence and Rohan's distress added to my self-loathing. I feared he wouldn't register a weight gain on his visits to the infant welfare center, and that the health sister would label me an unfit mother. Striving to eat only the right amounts of nutritional foods, I started a diet diary, telling myself that by stringently sticking to my rules, I would cope—but within two days another binge would occur.

Rohan was six weeks old when I had a severe binge. He vomited twice because I was upset, and that upset me further. The infant welfare nurse did not suspect a problem at his weigh-in, but I began to wean him to avoid the impact of further binges. They were difficult to avoid at the moment because George, wanting to be his own boss, was looking for a dairy farm to buy. At first I felt depressed and ate myself numb; then crawled out of the blackness, determined to make the most of yet another change, another fresh start. However, I was slipping and sliding into dark ravines. Each failure to settle caused my slips and slides to be steeper and more frequent than the one before.

1975: With a wonderful husband and three beautiful sons I felt depressed when, within a month, I resumed stuffing and starving myself. I was overflowing with milk one day and drying up the next. Somehow our new baby, Ben, coped admirably, and at night often slept twelve hours straight.

Oh, I am a silly billy. I ate like a horse all yesterday arvo till I felt quite sick. Now I am overflowing with milk! I only had a cup of tea for breakfast and I'm feeling better already. I'm going to go on the low carbohydrate diet, got to do something. I've started a health book and will buy a new set of bathroom scales this week; my present set have never been quite the same since my eldest son Shane put them in the bathwater.

1977: Four children under the age of five kept George and I busy, even with Council Home Help coming for several weeks after my tubal ligation operation. But being busy did not stop my niggling thoughts, and within weeks of Amanda's birth I began thinking about returning to work. The problem was to find someone capable of minding four children, the eldest of whom had yet to start preschool. With a gorgeous baby girl to love and hug, I felt silly to be talking about returning to work.

Emotionally my heart struggled to accept returning to work, but mentally I did not have a choice. My mood swings were such that George and my sister Joy together convinced me to return to work. The break from home would be good for the children and me and, although half my wage would go for childcare, every dollar was useful. Unemployment in Australia was twelve percent, the highest since World War Two.

I arranged to return to work at the start of April, giving myself time to wean Amanda and start a new diet in a bid to be free of depression, grumpiness and unhappiness. My many failed attempts to appease the tormentor in my mind were reducing my self-belief to rubble. I couldn't have any more babies, and dieting was not the answer. I had to clutch at something to raise myself out of the darkness, but I'd lost my way through fifteen years of dieting, each failure increasing my frustration and depression. Work was reassuring because, when I completed tasks and did a good job, I felt a little "normal."

1978: Building a new home, while living in it with four children under seven, had been a hard slog, but was easy compared with the struggle raging within me. Moving from place to place, which we did often (because my illness would not allow me to settle), and building a house was finite; it had a start and a finish. But my tormentor—a combination of eating disorder, depression and anxiety—was gray and black, an untouchable voracious mass in my mind:

I will get hold of myself one day. I hope I can do it without requiring special help. I figure it's probably me and my instability, insecurity that's caused us to have so many shifts, and probably my unhealthy, erratic, gluttonous diet that causes most of our arguments.

From my diary: *When I think of all the troubles in the world, mine are very small and I must overcome them before they destroy my life.*

The pressure of working eighteen-hour days to make the farm viable weighed heavily. I didn't need a husband for financial security, but I did need my husband for love and friendship, and lately George had no energy to give me either. Days passed without him saying "Good morning," let alone kiss me.

Increasingly I feared I was going around the bend, and thought I'd do our family and me a favor by seeing a psychologist. By most evenings, my head felt as delicate as a thin eggshell. Without any buffer, I screamed at the slightest provocation or noise. The sound of a child tapping a teaspoon on the table while waiting for dinner to be served resounded loudly in my brain and sent me running, holding my head, to the other end of the house. My tormentor thrived on such chaos. I called it a "tormentor" now, because at times I felt I could almost put my hand into my head and pull this dark, horrible mass out. My monster was becoming almost real, almost tangible. I began to think my instability and insecurity had caused our many shifts and arguments, and my tormentor wanted to destroy my marriage and my life. The shame and stigma were great, but my love for my children would give me strength to soon reach out, and share my inner hell of the past twenty years, with a doctor, for the first time.

*

OLIVIA ANTHONY
Olivia is a 44-year-old living
with anorexia nervosa and bulimia

I was successful at hiding my eating disorder at certain times in my life. I've also been very open about my eating disorders at different times. It depends on who the people are, too. If I feel safe and like I won't be judged for it, then I'll share. In college, when I slipped into bulimia, I was living with three other women. I isolated myself from them, which made me feel more alone in my illness. I polished off one of those big tubs of ice cream and kept it in my closet to use for purging. I ran the vacuum while purging to muffle the noises.

That summer I moved back home. There were six of us and there was only one bathroom, so I had to improvise. It's gross and embarrassing, but no ice cream bucket was big enough any longer. So I used big garbage bags to purge into and I kept them in my closet. I always posted a note on my door saying that I was working out, so basically leave me alone. I used that as an excuse for not answering the door while purging. It worked great until I was at work one day and my sister went to my closet to borrow something to wear. She found my purge bags. The smell most likely tipped her off. It's a miracle the bags never popped when I dragged them down the hallway in the mornings before work, to heave into the trunk. I drove to a park near my work and threw those bags into the dumpsters. After work that day my secret was out. My mom and sister were waiting for me at the kitchen table. My dad was in the family room, watching television. Mom and my sister told me they found the bags and also my journal. I couldn't believe they had read my journal. I felt so violated.

After I had my son, I relapsed when he was three. I told my friends and they were very supportive. They all helped care for Liam when I went for inpatient treatment, and also during my therapy and dietitian appointments. In 2011, I relapsed again but never told my family. I was ashamed and embarrassed to be struggling *again*. I didn't want to talk about it with any of them; I didn't want judgment from my sister.

*

CHRISTINE BASTONE
Christine is a 49-year-old living
with binge eating disorder

I don't really go to extremes to hide my eating disorder. I just don't binge in front of anybody. I'm never going to be the girl who eats just a salad, or just a little bit, in front of other people. I eat a lot in front of other people when there's food available, settings such as restaurants, parties, or having a meal at someone's house. I just don't binge later on that same day in front of them.

*

LYNDA CHELDELIN FELL
Lynda is a 50-year-old living
with binge eating disorder

Hiding binge eating is somewhat like hiding an alcohol addiction. I ate when nobody was looking. To make it look like I hadn't eaten so much, I simply baked another batch and pretended it was the first.

75

For a while I was fixated on a particular sandwich sold at a fast-food restaurant. I loved them, and almost couldn't eat enough. Mothering four children meant I ran lots of errands, so I always had an excuse to drive near that restaurant. Using the drive-thru meant I didn't have to get out of the car. I felt like a kid on Christmas morning, the anticipation of that "fix" was so strong. I always ordered the sandwich with an extra helping of sauce, and ate it before I exited the parking lot. Allowing the kids to order whatever they wanted distracted their attention from my fix. I never occurred to me that I might be setting them up to face the same beast. The goal was to get my fix before returning home, so my husband was none the wiser. Dinner was always cooked and served as if I hadn't eaten for hours. The secretiveness leads to shame, which leads to more eating to soothe the shame. It's a vicious cycle.

*

JUSTINE HILDEN
Justine is a 27-year-old living
with binge eating disorder

When I first was diagnosed with an eating disorder, I didn't tell people. I was embarrassed that I had an eating disorder when I ate significant amounts of food, and that I gained weight. I had thoughts such as "At least if I was anorexic, I would be skinnier," or "It would be better to be bulimic." They are crazy thoughts when I think back to it, but it was my reality. I was humiliated, embarrassed, and I just felt ashamed. It's as if I hoped no one would notice my weight gain, which only continued to go up and up.

I hid wrappers and containers, stopping at places to get rid of the evidence, eating dinner at home even though I had gone through a drive-thru on the way home, claiming I hadn't eaten when I had, and lying about what I had eaten. There was some adrenaline rush when I did these things. It was my little secret. No one knew about it but me.

As my mind became wiser, and my eating disorder voice became weaker, I have become more aware of just how ridiculous it all was. It doesn't happen as often, but it's there at times. I still hide wrappers or containers. There are times when I hit up dessert on the way home before I eat dinner. In the moments when I do, I feel good at first; the food makes me feel good, it's that initial "high." A burden is removed from my shoulder, and I just feel better. When I am eating, I feel calm, relaxed, all the problems of the day are gone. When I finish, I no longer feel calm or relaxed, and my problems are still there. It's a hard slap in the face. There is the guilt and the shame, which really feel just awful. The feelings of guilt and shame make me want to eat more and they make me feel terrible about myself.

*

LYDIA KENYON
Lydia is a 22-year-old living
with anorexia nervosa

I think my family knew before I did that I had something wrong with me. Whether they realized it was an eating disorder, or blamed depression throughout the whole process, there was really no hiding the truth from them...or was there? The ways I "hid" my behaviors were: pretending to eat when I wasn't, lying to my mom and hiding food, and lots of exercise. All these little tricks just helped to expedite my fear surrounding food. I continued to dabble in hurtful behaviors until September 2015, when I finally decided enough was enough and got on the road to recovery.

*

REBEKKAH KOONS
Rebekkah is a 29-year-old living with
eating disorder not otherwise specified

I waited for my roommates to go to sleep and then I would get my stash of food and chew and spit. Literally chew my food, spit it into a cup, and when the cup was full, flush the remains down the toilet. I hid eating disorder books throughout my room, and made sure I never went onto my eating disorder blog on a company computer. I didn't wear baggy clothes, because I wasn't ashamed at the time about my appearance; I thought I looked amazing when really I looked like a skeleton.

*

MONICA MIRKES
Monica is a 58-year-old living
with binge eating disorder

I hid treats, wait until everyone was asleep or gone, and then hurry to eat, not even enjoying the moment. I then felt guilty, but was not able to stop myself from continuing the behavior. I asked my husband to please not bring candy or snacks home. I would then find bags of M&Ms and other treats he brought home because they were on sale. I had no willpower. If it was there, I ate it.

*

RUTH PAPALAS
Ruth is a 58-year-old living
with binge eating disorder

I hid food I knew I shouldn't eat, and then eat it when no one was around. I even hid food from my family so I could have it all to myself. I threw wrappers into a dumpster or another place far away so no one would know I was eating what I shouldn't. I felt momentarily pleased that I got away with it. I would also feel ashamed knowing that I had even tried to get away with it, or mad because I felt like why shouldn't I eat whatever I want to? I also felt pleased that I succeeded in hiding it, but also knew it would show up later in my larger size. I'm a giant mess of emotions, and I eat my way through them.

*

DEBBIE PFIFFNER
Debbie is a 56-year-old living
with anorexia nervosa

Although I initially tried to hide it, my anorexia nervosa eventually became too obvious. As a student at a private school, I was required to wear a uniform consisting of a skirt, blouse, and vest or blazer. I couldn't hide the fact that my legs were sticks or my face was sunken. But I still tried to hide the fact that I wasn't eating. Since the school I attended did not have a hot lunch program, it was easy to walk by the trash can and toss my lunch, then tell everyone I wasn't hungry. Or go out with a friend and tell her I had eaten before I left home, and then tell my parents I had eaten when I was out. If someone asked whether I had eaten, I gave a great deal of latitude to that answer. After all, if I had a piece of candy, that meant I ate, didn't it? To me it did.

When my eating disorder came back twenty years later, I did try to hide it at first, but then quickly gave up. My family had already gone through this once before and knew the signs. My husband knew I had anorexia when I was younger, and he quickly became aware that something was wrong. Although he didn't completely understand what I was going through, he knew I needed help and support and he provided it for me. He did his best to support me while I was getting help and made sure that I knew he was proud of my accomplishments. My best friend was also extremely supportive. She is one of the very few people in my life with whom I can freely talk to about my disease and my fears. I know she will listen and not judge me. She may not have had an actual eating disorder, but she does her best to understand and support me. Recovery was easier this time because I knew I had people in my life who would understand my needs and support me, be my cheerleaders, and hold me up when I was beaten down.

*

DENISE PURCELL
Denise is a 50-year-old living
with anorexia nervosa and bulimia

I obsessively planned out meals in my head the day before. I couldn't take the chance of eating fat food. If I wasn't in control of my thoughts, I could easily binge alone in the bathroom late at night and then make myself throw up. I bought snacks and hid them, as well as the empty wrappers. I also hid the scales and weighed myself twice a day. When I started to look sickly, I hid myself under sweatshirts and long clothes. To others, there was no struggle. If I achieved what I should look like in their eyes, it was celebration enough that I was doing something right by not being fat. I always said my stomach hurt or that I ate earlier. I trained myself not to feel hungry and, in fact, not to feel anything at all.

*

HADDI TREBISOVSKY
Haddi is a 29-year-old living
with anorexia nervosa

There weren't many extremes I needed to carry out in order to conceal my eating disorder. I'm incredibly fortunate to never have been in grave danger regarding my anorexia, mainly because I didn't want to be caught and most of my meals were with family or friends who would have noticed if I stopped eating altogether. I skipped many lunches at school, where my parents couldn't see what I did or didn't eat. I could give reasonable excuses to my friends who wouldn't have known to look for clues at our age and season of life. When I got home, I would either binge on nachos and ice cream (I never purged) or continue my no-eating streak until dinner, depending on the day. I tried my best to balance these days out so that the binge days didn't undo my work from the restrictive days. As I restricted more frequently, I truly did feel satisfied with less food, and so I could say truthfully that I wasn't hungry anymore even if I had had only had a few bites of food. Again, I felt proud of the self-control that I thought I had, and at the same time I felt like I wasn't doing enough to punish myself.

*

The moment you accept yourself,
you become beautiful.
OSHO

*

CHAPTER FIVE

Fighting for Control

One of the reasons I was so unhappy for years was because I never embraced my emotions and I was trying to stay in control. -DEMI LOVATO

Control has a large role in most eating disorders, whether it be rigid control or the absence of any control. Whether it reflects a sense of mastery or failure, both reveal dysfunctional thinking patterns. How does control play a role in your eating disorder?

*

JUNE ALEXANDER
June is a 65-year-old living
beyond anorexia nervosa

The eating disorder fooled me into thinking that I was controlling me. However, in reality, the illness was controlling me and orchestrating a separation of self from body, causing me to engage in self-harming behaviors and thoughts, rather than actions and thoughts of self-love that are necessary for a healthy self and body connection. At age eleven, the same year anorexia developed, I received a diary as a gift. It marked the start of a literary journey in which the diary records the loss and recovery of self, and serves as a survival tool in both destructive and constructive ways.

Forty years would pass before recovery would enable me to be an observer as well as a participant in my experience and see how rules had aligned with, and fed, the eating disorder. I know now that there are only two things to remember in diary keeping: first, date each entry, and second, make no rules. I knew the first rule, but the second one eluded me. When you have an eating disorder, rules dominate every day, but they can be counterproductive. By age nineteen, pages of my diary were filling up with rules to live by. An eating disorder infiltrates thoughts and behavioral habits under the guise of helping to ease anxiety, control desires and manage self. It fools you into thinking it can help you be the person you want to be. It thrives on privacy—on a relationship with you alone—and encourages secrets. As a young woman, the diary presented to me as a safe place in which to sort thoughts, ease confusion, and practice self-control. But . . .

Confiding in the diary was also strengthening the eating disorder, where bossy demands became increasingly impossible to meet. When rules were inevitably broken, another punishing diet and exercise regime took their place. Nothing was ever enough.

By the time I was twenty-eight, the diary recorded an almost complete loss of self. Outwardly, I presented as a wife, mother, journalist, sister and daughter but within, the diary reveals a different story: of daily lists and pledges reflecting a desperate bid to stay sane and escape constant mental torment. A good day depended on strict adherence to my carefully crafted rules, set down in the diary, for instance, having to weigh this many pounds, run this many pounds, eat no more calories than this, and doing this, this and this…

I had been suffering an eating disorder for eighteen years when, feeling suicidal and fearing a diagnosis of madness, I shared the burden of my secret struggle with a doctor for the first time. The illness weakened my authentic self by creating secrets within secrets. Rational thought all but disappeared. My diary records the transformation from an honest, eager-to-please little girl to a shell of myself telling lies, not only to my mother ("Yes, I ate the sandwiches you packed for my lunch"), but also to myself. In fleeting moments of clarity, I was overcome with guilt and shame. The eating disorder fed on this, too, causing more isolation, more dependence, on perceived control and rules. Even when I became aware that the rules would fail, I continued to make them because I knew no other way of functioning and getting through each day. With the diary as keeper of eating disorder plans and schemes, lies to family, friends and self became more conniving and subversive. And out of control.

As years passed, the diary charted the secret toll of trying to function outwardly, while inwardly I was a slave to the eating disorder. So today, in recovery and continued healing, the word *control* has no place. Instead, my focus is on self-love, self-awareness and honing the *oneness* that comes with body and self integration. Read more about the diary as a self-help tool in my book, *Using Writing as a Therapy for Eating Disorders - The Diary Healer.*

*

OLIVIA ANTHONY
Olivia is a 44-year-old living
with anorexia nervosa and bulimia

For me, control played a huge part. When my weapon of abuse was anorexia, it helped me feel clean, safe, and secure. It made me feel like I was doing life right. I didn't have that anxiety corroding my brain. Whenever memories of past traumas invaded my thoughts, I counted the calories I'd eaten that day to help me focus on something I was in control of. As I watched my body shrinking, I felt safer. I felt in control. But I wasn't in control, really, and I did know that on some level. The last time I relapsed, my body couldn't take it like it used to. I could see that I was killing my body, and I knew I was out of control. But I couldn't stop restricting. When I turned away food and still stayed alive, it made me feel powerful! I felt like I was completely in control. When my body fought back and drove me to eat, bulimia took over. I felt really out of control during the binges.

In college, after an empty ice cream bucket in my bedroom would no longer suffice for purging into, I left my apartment to use the science building's bathrooms. On the walk over, I had intense anxiety, worrying about all the calories sitting in my stomach. Immediately after purging I felt immense relief. It was also like a high. I felt clean. I felt in control again. But it didn't take long before life's issues invaded, or I got hungry, and the whole cycle started again. Also, I think control played a part in that I felt so unsure of what my purpose on this Earth was. I didn't really know what to do with life. It felt out of control. But I was able to control what I ate or whether or not I kept food.

*

CHRISTINE BASTONE
Christine is a 49-year-old living
with binge eating disorder

I don't feel like I have any control in my eating disorder. I feel very out of control. I can't stop myself from eating too much, can't stop myself from bingeing. I very much wish that I had even partial control when it comes to eating. That would be a big improvement.

*

LYNDA CHELDELIN FELL
Lynda is a 50-year-old living
with binge eating disorder

Control? I had no control. It was terrible. In addition, I never felt satiated, never felt full. No matter how much I ate, my body lacked the natural ability to signal that I had taken in far more calories than my body could use. As a result, my portion sizes were enormous. Add a second or third helping, and I might feel full momentarily, but it passed quickly. My brother, who was two years older, was an athlete and could eat huge portions and multiple helpings and remain thin. My seat at the dinner table was next to his, so my perception of portion size was skewed.

Magazines, movies, and television depict mostly skinny women. I often fantasized about what it might feel like to never to worry about one's weight. The lives of skinny women seem so carefree and idyllic. I wanted to be thin, too. In my mind, thin meant a life without problems. But of course that is akin to the poor who believe that all their worldly problems would be solved if only they had money.

When something feels out of reach, we think that *if only* is the magic cure. If only I were skinny. If only I were rich.

While growing up, the emphasis was always on size: pant sizes, bra sizes, shirt sizes, and dress sizes. Even our pantyhose size was scrutinized. Although the size charts weren't realistic, the clothing labels trumped: size ten/twelve is the same as size Large. How humiliating! In our culture, fat is synonymous with ugly. The feeling of never measuring up to what society deems beautiful prompted me to seek even more comfort in...what else?....food. Oh, how I envied those girls who were skinny. I was sure they hadn't a worry in the world. Now that I've been thin for ten years, I can see that being a healthy weight doesn't fix life's problems. My life isn't carefree nor idyllic. Maybe that is why I'm passionate about speaking out....so others don't feel so alone.

*

LYDIA KENYON
Lydia is a 22-year-old living
with anorexia nervosa

I used to firmly believe that control did *not* play any sort of role. I know now that it is in fact a huge part of the anorexia. I can pinpoint a moment when I felt out of control completely, and turned to restricting (albeit unknowingly) at that time. Sadly, that control issue has stayed with me, and eating less did take care of what I lacked control over.

THROUGH THE EYES OF AN EATING DISORDER

*

REBEKKAH KOONS
Rebekkah is a 29-year-old living with
an eating disorder not otherwise specified

Control was a small part of my eating disorder. I used it mostly to cope with the grief and loneliness that I felt all the time. The only time I felt in control was when I was hurting my family, and I knew they couldn't do anything to stop me. They knew this, and didn't try very hard, but it gave me a sense of identity in my family, I had a "thing" I was good at. Coming from a large family, I always felt invisible. But my eating disorder made me more visible than I had ever been.

*

RUTH PAPALAS
Ruth is a 58-year-old living
with binge eating disorder

Control is hard, because I can control almost every other area of my life. What I can't seem to control is my desire to eat or my seemingly endless hunger. I eat sometimes to get the offending food out of the house; I can't just waste it by throwing it away. I eat it all and then think, "Good, now I'll be okay." Then I go buy more because it was on sale, or it was good and I haven't had that for a long time. So it starts all over again. It's quite a vicious cycle.

*

DEBBIE PFIFFNER
Debbie is a 56-year-old living
with anorexia nervosa

Control plays is big role in my eating disorder. I have heard it said many times that eating disorders can be the result of feeling that

89

everything in your life is out of your control, and eating or not eating is one thing that only you can control. I believe that statement. My life has been a constant stream of things that I have no control over, but I always have control over what I put in my body. That's my choice— my decision, and you can't force me to eat. Even if you could, I would find a way to purge or starve myself to show that I was the one in control, not you. There have also been times when I've felt totally out of control. I wanted to be normal. I really did. But the eating disorder had control over me, and I literally could not get out from underneath that control. Now I'm starting to let that control go and to acknowledge that there are just some things I will never be able to control. I will never be normal, but I can be healthy—both physically and mentally. That is most important.

*

DENISE PURCELL
Denise is a 50-year-old living
with anorexia nervosa and bulimia

For me it's both. I have no control over my own feelings or behaviors because of my past, so it's never somewhere in the middle or gray area. It's always extreme. So when I feel like I'm in control, I binge or overeat. When I feel no control, I punish and don't eat, or eat and purge. The fight will never go away; it's an addiction cycle. Sometimes I win, sometimes I lose. But I'm never really the winner, because I will never be happy with the way I look or feel. It's a vicious cycle.

*

HADDI TREBISOVSKY
Haddi is a 29-year-old living
with anorexia nervosa

During the years I battled with my ED, I felt very in control over my eating, and it gave me a sense of pride because I felt that it was more an avenue of discipline rather than an unhealthy relationship with control. Looking back, however, I realize that my sense of control came from a deep need to define myself as "the skinny girl." I had always been thin as a girl, and somewhere along the way I became fearful of gaining weight. I felt it was necessary to stay as thin as possible in order to be the Haddi everyone knew and expected. My image was everything to me, and I felt that if I lost control over my image I wouldn't know who I was anymore, and I wouldn't be able to find worth in that girl.

*

There is no magic cure,
no making it all go away forever.
There are only small steps upward;
an easier day, an unexpected laugh,
a mirror that doesn't matter anymore.
LAURIE HALSE ANDERSON

*

CHAPTER SIX

Shame and Blame

Some say that a flaw is unacceptable. Grace
says that though I am flawed, I am cherished.
-ANONYMOUS

The dictionary defines shame as a painful feeling of humiliation or distress caused by the consciousness of wrong or foolish behavior. Whether one believes that shame results from the eating disorder, or is to blame for the eating disorder, the role it plays is undeniable. How does shame influence your eating disorder?

*

JUNE ALEXANDER
June is a 65-year-old living with
beyond anorexia nervosa

Secrecy and shame dominated my disorder for more than four decades. I had no sense of pride from being "successful." I did have a feeling of being able to cope and manage life on the rare days when I managed to abide by the secret lists of rules set the day before.

There are many types of secrets; they vary in nature and origin. For example, there can be family secrets, and then there is the secret within, of the eating disorder, which masquerades as a personal, trustworthy friend. There is no place for any type of secret in healing from an eating disorder. Everything must be in the open to avoid the ED twisting and manipulating the secret to enforce isolation.

Dealing with the fallout of exposed secrets, those of which you are aware or suspect they exist, can be painful enough. But there can be more sinister secrets, those of which you are not consciously aware. An eating disorder can be in this elusive category. Initially you may feel some unease, that something's not right, and have a feeling of emptiness that cannot be addressed. But there is no helpful sign saying LOOK OUT or SEEK GUIDANCE NOW. ED can sneak into your mind and your behavioral habits under the guise of helping to ease anxiety, control desires and manage yourself. It can fool you into thinking it can help you be the person you want to be. This silent bully thrives on privacy, on its relationship with you alone, and encourages secrets. Its entry is so subtle and contrived that you might not recognize the illness thoughts, which first appear trustworthy, friendly and intimate, but then become omnipresent, all powerful, and aren't the real you.

For healing to occur, secrets related to ED must be disclosed, or at least acknowledged, and dealt with honestly. Truth with oneself must reign. If queried during my illness, I would have strenuously insisted my diary harbored no secrets, especially from me. It was my friend and confidant, after all. But the harsh truth was that the illness that invaded my mind also sabotaged my diary.

My secrets developed slowly. I progressively withdrew, and ED went from strength to strength. The illness weakened me by creating secrets within secrets. With ED's "support," I transformed from an honest, eager-to-please little girl to a shell of myself, telling lies not only to my mother (for example, insisting that I ate the sandwiches she packed for my school lunch, when I had given them to playmates or thrown them away), but most of all, to myself. In fleeting moments of clarity, I felt overcome with guilt. My eating disorder fed on this, increasing its dominance over my will and bullying my thoughts.

My mother spent hours preparing favorite meals, and I refused to eat them. One day, as a special holiday treat, on an outing to town, she bought a soft vanilla ice cream in a cone for me and, as soon as her back was turned, I dropped it in the street gutter. She turned, seeing what had had happened, and was dismayed. Filled with shame, I muttered, "Oh, sorry. It slipped." Oh, what was this thing that was making me do things I did not want to do, that was causing my loved ones so much distress? It was the eating disorder, of course, but I would not find help for another twenty years, by which time my mother had lost sight of the little girl who was.

Today I am a grandmother, and I have no secrets. My life is an open book, to the extent that my young grandchildren sit beside me while I write in my diary, and often ask if they can add a few words too. I always say yes, for my story is also their story. No secrets, no shame, no stigma. For more insights about the impact of secrets, see chapter four in my book *Using Writing as a Therapy for Eating Disorders - The Diary Healer*.

*

OLIVIA ANTHONY
Olivia is a 44-year-old living
with anorexia nervosa and bulimia

While married to my eating disorder, I isolated myself. Depression was also part of it. I remember going to a party that some Norwegian students invited me to. They were the kindest people, and I have only positive memories of them. But the whole time I was there I was thinking about pop tarts! I wanted to go home and binge and purge up pop tarts. Mostly ED was my main companion. I looked forward to spending time with ED more than anything. As the years passed, that relationship changed, though. I felt a lot more shame over what I was doing to my son's mother. What would he do if I died? I felt horrible thinking about that. My love for my son was what drove me to fight for my life.

*

CHRISTINE BASTONE
Christine is a 49-year-old living
with binge eating disorder

I think that shame affects my eating disorder by driving me to eat more. Unfortunately, it's a vicious circle. Otherwise I'm not sure. I don't believe that my shame about my eating disorder influences my daily routine, though. This is probably because I am isolated a lot of the time, since I am a stay-at-home mom, and most weekdays I spend a number of hours at home alone while my family is at work or school.

*

LYNDA CHELDELIN FELL
Lynda is a 50-year-old living
with binge eating disorder

The feelings of shame colored every aspect of my life. I questioned my worth to my husband, my family, and even society. Did my husband find me sexy? Were my kids embarrassed? When I was fat, people in society ignored me. I remember desperately wanting to be viewed as having some sense of worth. But books are unequivocally judged by the cover. Obesity carries double stigmas of low intelligence and laziness. Feeling ashamed for having such a large size is compounded by having to work harder to prove our worth. Add in the frequent looks of disgust by the waitress, or the traveler when he discovers his seat is next to an obese person, and you might understand why we are filled with shame. We could be a rocket scientist or a brilliant entrepreneur, but the fat person will always be the last person picked for a team. True story.

Now that I'm thin, I'm treated in a drastically different way. People look me in the eye and listen when I speak. They pay attention, confident that I have something valuable to say. My voice is no different than it was, but society holds me with more regard now that I'm thin. I might be half my size, but I'm still me. After having experienced both sides of the coin, I feel a tremendous amount of empathy for what the obese face in public. On one end of the spectrum, they are invisible and ignored. On the other end, they are treated rudely, bullied and harassed. And nobody steps in. Nobody. Because it appears that we brought the problem on ourselves.

*

LYDIA KENYON
Lydia is a 22-year-old living
with anorexia nervosa

I used to feel so ashamed, and told my mom not to let my brother and sisters know what I had. At some point, it seemed as though everyone knew, or they suspected. I slowly began to open up, mostly on social media and through starting a blog. Now I am no longer as ashamed about my health issues. They are what they are, and I am trying to get better. I think that there is so much shame and secrecy because eating disorders are still a mental illness that isn't talked about as much. Talk about it. If it is talked about, it becomes less of a secret.

*

REBEKKAH KOONS
Rebekkah is a 29-year-old living with an
eating disorder not otherwise specified

I felt ashamed only if I got caught in an eating disorder act. If I got away with it, then I did have a sense of pride and I'd use that feeling to get my mind set to succeed with other things in my life.

*

RUTH PAPALAS
Ruth is a 58-year-old living
with binge eating disorder

My daily routine is a mix of eating and trying to hide my size in clothes. Every night when I go to bed, I swear that tomorrow will be the day when I'm going to start losing weight again. I *will* eat healthy. I *will not* overeat. I wake up *knowing* today is the day. Then life happens. I get a phone call, text, an unexpected bill in the mail...it doesn't take much to send me seeking out a perfect combination of salty and sweet or maybe an extra savory treat. After I come out of my feeding frenzy, the reality of what I've done *again* hits me. The feelings of guilt and shame stress me out, and I start all over again. I always wonder why I can't stop myself. My head knows better. I eat to feed a feeling, an emotion—not because I'm stomach hungry.

I read somewhere that when you eat to fill a void, you're craving a specific food and only that food will meet your needs. When you eat because you're hungry, you're open to options. Many times I am not open to options. I have a tendency to think I feel hungry intensely and all of a sudden, instead of gradually. I crave junk foods. My urge to eat is usually preceded by stress or an uncomfortable emotion such as sadness, anger, boredom, guilt or frustration. And the cycle starts all over again.

*

DEBBIE PFIFFNER
Debbie is a 56-year-old living
with anorexia nervosa

When my eating disorder first began and in the years that followed, I would say there was more secrecy and shame involved than there is for me now. There were many social activities that I avoided that involved food. I did not want to eat in front of people. It was easy to say that I ate enough, but if people saw what I really was eating, they would know I was not eating normally. I came very close to losing a friendship because my friend was extremely vocal about me not eating enough. It got to the point where I didn't want to be around her, because she brought it up all the time and she didn't really understand what I was going through. A lot of times, if there was a social activity that involved dinner or eating, I would just avoid it totally.

I felt ashamed that although I knew my eating disorder was not a good thing, and that I was slowly killing myself, I couldn't do anything about it. I wanted to be skinny. I did not want to gain weight. People would stare at me, and, although they were staring at me because of the awful way my body looked, it felt good to have people looking. And then I felt ashamed for feeling that way.

My feelings of secrecy and shame have changed over the years. I no longer let my eating disorder dictate what social activities I will attend. I no longer isolate myself. I have a good support system, and people know that my eating disorder is an issue I am working hard to overcome. I no longer feel proud when someone stares at me. If someone does, my standard response is to smile and wave. That makes them aware that I know they are watching me, and they usually look away. And since I know I'm getting better, I don't feel ashamed. There is no secrecy attached anymore. I was shopping recently when a woman said, "Oh, my God! You have one of them eating disorders, don't you? You should leave here and go to Burger King and eat one of them Whoppers. That will fatten you up." Years ago, that might have made me feel good, and then ashamed for feeling good. But when this happened, all I did was smile at the woman and say "Okay, thanks," and then grabbed my cart and moved on. I knew where I was in my disease and recovery, and that's all that mattered.

*

DENISE PURCELL
Denise is a 50-year-old living
with anorexia nervosa and bulimia

I don't ever feel pride. If I'm on the skinnier side of things, I have a false sense of satisfaction. But it never stops the cycle I'm on. I'm ashamed that I feel this way, that I can't accept myself no matter what. I base my everyday decisions on what other people think of me. That sends me into a spiral. Healthy would be great, though I don't know what that is. All I know is that fat and ugly is unacceptable, and I should hide from the world. Skinny means you are pretty and accepted, even if you're not happy.

*

HADDI TREBISOVSKY
Haddi is a 29-year-old living
with anorexia nervosa

I no longer struggle with anorexia, but when I was actively struggling I was very secretive and felt full of shame not only for the way I was handling things, but also for the way I looked. I felt shameful if I noticed that my tummy was softer than I liked, for example. After getting free from my eating disorder, I found that it's very important for me to get ahead of relapse by sharing even the slightest insecurities with my husband or others in my support system. They are able to talk me through my feelings and help me to rationalize my emotions before I get a chance to put my insecurities into action by skipping meals. In essence, I've realized that the best way to combat the power that secrecy and shame might have over me is to expose them.

I am forever engaged in a silent battle in my
Head over whether or not to lift the fork to my
mouth, and when I talk myself into doing so, I
taste only shame. I have an eating disorder.
JENA MORROW

*

CHAPTER SEVEN

The Self Esteem Influence

Movies can and do have a tremendous influence in shaping young lives in the realm of entertainment towards the ideals and objectives of normal adulthood. -WALT DISNEY

Self-esteem, identity, and body image are closely related in developing adolescents. They are also deeply woven into the fabric of eating disorders, yet remain one of the biggest challenges of recovery. How does your eating disorder influence your identity?

*

JUNE ALEXANDER
June is a 65-year-old living
beyond anorexia nervosa

The eating disorder had a great influence on my identity and self-esteem because it developed at age eleven. When parts of childhood, adolescence and young adulthood slip by while entrapped in a mental illness or debilitated by trauma, there is much life learning and experience to catch up on. Under the guidance of a psychiatrist who recognized the value of the narrative as a recovery tool, my diaries became teachers, helping me to let go of rules and discover and experience life as *me*. Re-awakening of self was a tenuous process, with the diary chronicling the gradual change from living by the eating disorder's impossible rules to locating, embracing, and learning to express and have faith in true thoughts and feelings.

Tentatively, driven by an urge to learn more about the illness that had profoundly affected my life and that of my loved ones, in 2009, at the age of fifty-eight, I began to attend eating disorder conferences. There I was at the first such event —a sufferer, and by now a grandmother, among all these highly professional and respected people. I felt nervous and out of place, until the researchers stood behind the lectern to describe their latest findings. Then I sat entranced, on the edge of my seat, wanting to call out in elation, "You are describing my life; you are helping me understand me." Their words illuminated my mind. They helped me accept that I was an okay person. I began to feel I belonged. I had had an illness that had made me feel worthless, that was all.

Sadly, efforts to reunite with my family of origin failed. My parents and sister had labeled me the only one with a problem in the family, and for many years I believed them. Now, however, I could see that an eating disorder affected every member of the family. I wanted to show my parents and sister that the little girl they knew and loved all those years ago had been present all the time, suppressed by the illness. I continued to seek family unity and acceptance. But perhaps too much time had passed, for they made a life that did not include me.

My children's dad accompanied me to both of my parents' funerals, in 2009 and 2010. As we departed the church from the second funeral, he said, "Now you are free. Our children and our grandchildren are your family. Focus on them." His words were true, and healing continued in unexpected ways. The black and white of my father's will, for instance, backed what my carers and treatment team had been saying. In a bittersweet way this formal, legal notification enhanced my freedom. I hadn't imagined the rejection after all. It was real. It was of their doing. I did not deserve to be punished. I was not a bad person. I was free to move on.

It is tough, awfully tough, getting out of the anorexic prison with your life but without your childhood family, which was my experience. I cope by counting blessings. I'm sure my parents loved me, but they didn't know how to cope. I had to change, to live, but they had become comfortable in their groove.

I owe my life to a network of support that includes my children's dad, my children and grandchildren, friends, psychiatrist, therapists, doctors, neurosurgeon, minister of religion and faith in God. While I became alienated from my family of origin, and lost my marriage, I have gained another family in recovery—a family comprising people from all walks of life in the eating disorder field. This family of choice nurtures my fledgling self-belief. Acknowledging the person before the illness, and respecting the person beyond the illness, makes a world of difference. Respect gives hope.

Today, anorexia nervosa has been replaced with the joy and love of family, self and life. I awaken each day with a sense of purpose. For instance, experience in healing from an eating disorder after more than forty years led me to become a Ph.D. candidate at age sixty-five. Writing has enabled the re-storying of hurtful, traumatic experiences in a way that allows me to embrace the current moment. The passion for writing that helped me to survive privately has become a sword in fighting eating disorders around the world, by disseminating evidence-based research.

Love, three nutritious meals and three snacks a day, together with walks by the seashore, are my maintenance program. I'll never know if I am the person I would have been had I not developed anorexia nervosa at age eleven. What I do know is that I am free. My life is not wasted. My life has purpose: as a mother, grandmother, writer and advocate. Most precious of all, I am me and I am happy with me.

*

OLIVIA ANTHONY
Olivia is a 44-year-old living
with anorexia nervosa and bulimia

I spent years believing that I was nothing but an anorexic or bulimic. I believed that there was nothing else that I was good at. That there was nothing else to me. I thought that I was a huge waste of space and that the world would be better off without me. When I had my son and was remarried to my eating disorder, I didn't identify as strongly with believing I was only an anorexic/bulimic. I saw myself as mommy and I wanted to divorce ED so much. I have felt so hopeless and powerless each time I was entrenched in it. It's so hard to not listen to that ED voice that is telling you how awful you are. On the flip side of that, in the beginning when I was just starting to slip down that slippery slope, I felt so great! I remember feeling relieved that I would never have to worry about getting fat. I held the magical key to that! I felt really good and powerful. It didn't take long to get depressed, though. It was such a prison and it felt like a life sentence. It made me ultimately feel like a loser.

*

CHRISTINE BASTONE
Christine is a 49-year-old living
with binge eating disorder

My eating disorder has had an extremely negative effect on my self-esteem. Being out of control, especially about something as basic as eating, is not kind to someone's self-esteem. I used to be skinny, but that was a very, very long time ago. Now I am fat, and there's no getting away from it. Of course, I have to take my body with me everywhere I go! Every time I look in the mirror, every time I try to figure out what to wear, every time I take a bath, every time I adjust my clothes to keep my belly from showing, even every time I read my Kindle or play a game on my tablet, I am reminded and disgusted by what I look like.

*

LYNDA CHELDELIN FELL
Lynda is a 50-year-old living
with binge eating disorder

My binge eating and obesity had a severe impact upon my self-esteem. I am the third of four daughters and countless times I heard my mother say, "She would be so pretty if only she lost weight." This comment wasn't reserved just for family; it was applied to strangers too. So in my skewed thinking, only thin girls were pretty. And being pretty solved everything. Looking back, I now understand that my mother's generation believed that a child's behavior was a direct reflection of their own success as a parent. When a child misbehaved, the mother was faulted for poor parenting. But if a child succeeded, the parents were given the glory. This thinking also applied to physical appearance. An obese daughter brought shame to the mother. Words can heal, or words can harm. My mother's tongue was razor sharp.

Taught to believe that only thin girls were pretty, I tried every diet under the sun. And failed every time. The repeated failures led not only to my mother's shame, but to my own as well. Why couldn't I stop with just one cookie or one enchilada? Not only did the obesity affect my self-esteem, but so did the shame from lack of control. The cycle was vicious and felt endless.

Over the years, I've succeeded in shedding one hundred pounds three different times. In my search for improved self-worth, my answer was to severely restrict my dietary intake while exercising. But that, too, was extreme. At one point I was exercising three hours a day. I never learned to master an even keel. The result was that each time I shed the weight, I became too thin. And then I heard, "Don't lose too much weight or you'll be all wrinkly, like your Aunt Darling." I just couldn't win. Consequently, I spent a good deal of my life trying to please others instead of getting to know myself. My self-esteem was always low. I used food for my reward, punishment, or both.

Just as addicts like to hang out with addicts, dieting was all inclusive in our family of girls. Our only brother was athletic and naturally thin. But we girls, in Mom's eyes, could always stand to lose a few pounds. Mom and Dad married in the 1950s, and our family was classic of the times. Dad was a white-collar mechanical engineer. Mom stayed home to raise us five kids. We lacked for nothing, and had a good, stable childhood. But if Mom decided she was getting too heavy, us girls could "stand to lose a few pounds" too. At size ten, I soon found myself at the mercy of Slim-Fast, the Beverly Hills Diet, the Scarsdale Diet, and Jane Fonda.

My quest for self-esteem was found solely in my weight. I never learned balance. And I always let others direct my helm.

*

LYDIA KENYON
Lydia is a 22-year-old living
with anorexia nervosa

I definitely feel like I have related myself and the eating disorder to one being. One of the things I have done in therapy is to separate the two. I have now named the eating disorder "Ed." It is so much easier now to see what Ed says, and what I say, and how they differ. I used to get so frustrated because my mom told me, "That's not you, that's the eating disorder talking." In some ways that was true. But in saying that, I began to get angry because it seemed no one would listen to *me* anymore.

As I began recovery, I would anxiously ponder who I was now. I wasn't the skinniest one in the room. I would no longer be the girl who didn't eat. Slowly and surely I am finding my way. What you eat or don't eat doesn't have to define you, and neither does your size.

*

REBEKKAH KOONS
Rebekkah is a 29-year-old living with
an eating disorder not otherwise specified

I've always been the small, tiny girl. I loved the jokes about how small I was, etc. When I was at my heaviest, I didn't even know who I was. It wasn't me, and I hated every second of it to the point where I didn't even want to get out of bed. When I finally lost about twenty pounds, it was the mental weight being lifted as well, and I was Rebekkah again.

*

RUTH PAPALAS
Ruth is a 58-year-old living
with binge eating disorder

As a married adult, I was always Mike's mom, Breanne's mom, or Nick's wife, or Dave and Judy's daughter. I often wondered if it was an embarrassment for them to introduce me due to my size. There are times when I still wonder if they think, "I wish she would lose some weight and keep it off." I ponder the same thing myself.

I avoided the beach and swimming pools until I was about forty years old. I didn't want to be seen in a swimsuit. When I was invited on the trip of a lifetime to Jamaica (after my gastric bypass) I still didn't feel my body was beach worthy, but I *had* to go! It was my first time! I went and had a great time. For the very first time in my life, I realized I would never be the best looking one on the beach. I will also never be the worst looking one on the beach. That is also my advice to anyone who is afraid to be seen on a beach due to their size: You'll never be the best or the worst on the beach. Go and have fun. I also have to admit that when I get to the beach, I actually look for someone who is larger than me. Sad, but I secretly say "Thank you for being here today." Sometimes I'm able to get over myself, and other times it's a struggle.

*

DEBBIE PFIFFNER
Debbie is a 56-year-old living
with anorexia nervosa

Since my eating disorder has been a part of my life for the better part of forty years, I would say my eating disorder has been my identity. My family, friends and anyone who knew me knew I had an eating disorder. They knew I was too thin, and that my eating habits were weird.

A few years back, I conducted an experiment with the girls I worked with. I gave them all a piece of paper and asked them, without thinking about it, to write down what they would say to someone who needed to find me in a crowded place. The consensus was "the tall, really skinny blonde." That was my identity. I didn't know it was happening until someone referred to me that way. My eating disorder became who I was. I was an anorexic. I don't believe there is anything really positive about being defined that way, but I think I will always be thought of in that way by my family. Does it bother me? Yes and no. It bothers me that weight defines anyone. But I try not to let it get to me. As long as I know my truth, that needs to be enough.

I have never really had much self-esteem. Did the eating disorder affect it? I don't clearly see that it did affect my self-esteem either positively or negatively. I had a self-esteem problem long before I developed the eating disorder, and it's possible that developing the eating disorder may have had to do with my lack of self-esteem. As I grow as a person, and receive more and more support from some unexpected sources, my self-esteem increases, and maybe one day I will not be defined by my eating disorder.

*

DENISE PURCELL
Denise is a 50-year-old living
with anorexia nervosa and bulimia

Sadness comes up for me. It has defined me and I allowed it; not willingly, but I learned how the game works. Back when I was twenty, fifty seemed so old. I always said that when I turn fifty, that I was going to eat what I want and be happy no matter what, because I earned it.

Well, I'm fifty. And yes, I've completely gone toward the bingeing side, but not always. I hate the way I look. There is no positive in eating disorders. The only thing I can do is be honest with my girls, and tell them to deal with their feelings; be who they are at all times. Because our body is forever changing. It's not your size or the color of your hair, it's who you are inside and your values and strengths. The kindness and compassion you show to people, and forever being humble. Life is too short to be fixated on such things as these. Maybe a different generation and a way of thinking, a way of being aware of how we treat and talk and teach our young, will be the foundation for them to grow. So let's be strong and teach them not to do as we have, but to be strong in themselves.

*

HADDI TREBISOVSKY
Haddi is a 29-year-old living
with anorexia nervosa

While I was actively struggling, my eating disorder absolutely helped me to shape the identity I wanted for myself. I didn't necessarily think of myself as a girl with ED, but more as a thin girl who would always remain thin because she had control over the situation. I didn't acknowledge how unhealthy this thought process was for a few years. I simultaneously had great AND awful self-esteem. I was happy when people commented on how thin I was. But when I studied myself too long, or thought about how I looked compared to other thin girls, my self-esteem would fall. For a long time, my identity was wrapped up in the way I looked and how much I weighed.

Now that I'm free of ED's bondage, I view ED as part of my story, and while I wouldn't say that it defines me or my identity today, it's a part of who I was and am. Because of that, I live my life a little differently than others do. Because I know that I've been prone to an ED in the past, I take precautions that others don't have to think about. I don't own a scale, I never skip meals even if I don't feel like eating, and if the slightest hint of insecurity comes up, I address it immediately with a trusted person so she can give me the support I need before I slip back into the darkness of the ED (or depression or anxiety, depending on what the trigger is). In this way, ED has shaped a part of my life, but I'm grateful for all the ways I've learned to be stronger through my healing.

Clouds come floating into my life, no
longer to carry rain or usher storm,
but to add color to my sunset sky.
RABINDRANATH TAGORE

*

CHAPTER EIGHT

Domino Effect on Health

Health is a state of complete physical, mental, and social well-being, and not merely the absence of disease or infirmity. -WORLD HEALTH ORGANIZATION

Although eating disorders are considered a mental illness, the physical effects cannot be ignored, and they increase over time. Anorexia and bulimia deny the body of essential nourishment, and can lead to long-term damage and even death. Binge eating disorder results in excessive caloric intake, which can lead to diabetes, hypertension, high cholesterol, and arthritis. Has your eating disorder affected your physical health, and if so, how?

*

JUNE ALEXANDER
June is a 65-year-old living
beyond anorexia nervosa

My eating disorder's effects on my physical health have been wide-ranging, starting in childhood and continuing for the next four decades. Also, due to the longevity of my eating disorder, even when free of its symptoms, the biological effects of the illness have continued to present health challenges.

I began to menstruate a week or so after my eleventh birthday. My mother had not forewarned me or explained anything about periods. Anorexia developed within six months of the start of menstruation. Eventually, the monthly period petered out to an occasional period, and then none at all. So that was one effect on my physical health. I had other effects like lanugo, swollen ankles, sores on my fingers that wouldn't heal—all signs of malnutrition and starvation. These effects were more short term, and were overcome when my anorexia transitioned to bulimia tendencies.

But my periods had not resumed by age fifteen and my mother, feeling concerned, took me to a doctor who prescribed a birth control pill. The first attempt of three months failed to resume my menstruation, so I had to take the medication for another six months. This time it worked. I became buxom and gained xxx kilograms in fourteen weeks. Everyone thought I was normal.

At age twenty, I fainted on the morning of my wedding. I fainted regularly. Ten weeks after the wedding, I binged on ten scones one morning before driving to the newspaper office where I was a cadet reporter. Lacking concentration, my mind foggy and full of self-loathing from stuffing myself with food, I drove under a loaded log truck and sustained cervical spine injuries. My husband George always said, "You weren't the same after that accident." Mood swings and headaches increased. Several decades would pass before a neurosurgeon said, "I believe I can help you, and take away ninety percent of your pain." Doctors said I had been one-sixteenth of an inch from snapping my spine, so I had been fortunate. The eating disorder had almost driven me to my death.

Pregnancies provided another health challenge. My first was not planned. I was in the third year of my journalism cadetship, and had not thought about having a baby. Now that I was pregnant, however, I proceeded to give birth to four children within four years. Having babies became a way of creating a milepost, a defined period: each pregnancy gave nine months to get myself in order, to stop bingeing, eat normally, to be free of torment.

My diary, 1976: *I can have xxx calories per day until Bubsie comes, then xxxx, only increasing if weight falls below xxx, and decreasing if above xxx six weeks after Bubsie's birth.*

But within a week of each birth, the binge-starve cycle became worse than before. Five months into the third pregnancy, acute appendicitis required an emergency operation. Early in the fourth pregnancy, I almost lost the baby. My body lacked iron, among other things. The gynecologist said he was not worried about the baby being small, but about it starving. He didn't ask about nutrition and didn't know about my rollercoaster eating patterns or dark moods. Four weeks prior to my due date, the doctor said, "What a scungy kid you've got in there." His words stung, but because he was the only doctor who performed the tubal ligation operation, I had to remain his patient.

At some level, I knew I could not go on having babies. I was the major breadwinner, continuing to maintain employment at a time when many people frowned upon working mothers, and the only way to stop this pattern of having babies was to have a tubal ligation before returning home with baby number four. However, the tubal ligation would also prevent my use of pregnancy as a lever to fight my tormentor, and this worried me. Now that the baby option was eliminated, descent into chronic depression and anxiety was swift.

At age twenty-eight, deep love for my four young children drove me to share what were by now suicidal thoughts and actions with a doctor for the first time. Four years of misdiagnosis followed. The first doctor said my brain had a gap or deficiency, which affected large brain messages having to do with mood, memory, self-esteem, and so on. Possibly a lack of oxygen to my brain had occurred in the few hours before I was born. He wrote a prescription for pills and said "You will be a new person." No, I felt worse. He referred me to a clinical psychologist who probed a little farther, diagnosed chronic hypoglycemia, and provided a special diet. The psychologist also prescribed vitamins and minerals at ten times the normal dosage. He concluded that I ate because I was deprived and felt unloved, that the basic problem was my marriage, and suggested I needed more hugs.

I tried to believe the hypoglycemia diet was helping, but I was fooling the psychologist and myself. All the while the symptoms were getting more severe. Repetitive sounds, like a child tapping a teaspoon on the table while waiting for dinner, drove me crazy; my head felt as fragile as an egg without a shell. There was no point trying to discuss any of this with my family, because their standard response was, "You think too much," and "Think about others instead of yourself."

In my forties, two operations provided important recovery steps. One was a hysterectomy; I had already experienced menopause. The other was the insertion of a six centimeter titanium rod, buttressed each end in my cervical spine from C4 to T1. Four discs and three vertebrae were removed. Twenty-seven years after colliding with the log truck, medical advances had enabled this life-changing operation.

In my fifties, diagnosis of Hashimoto's disease, an autoimmune condition, marked another step in the rebuilding of self. Ongoing medication for this condition helped considerably in advancing general feelings of wellness and addressing auto-immune deficiencies.

In a development that science suggests may be related to the thyroid condition, in my sixties I have begun to experience recurring bouts of chronic urticaria. By some miracle, and largely due to caring dentists, I still have my own teeth. I like to think that my early childhood on a family dairy farm, drinking lots of fresh, warm cows' milk before developing anorexia, has held me in good stead, and my bones have managed to avoid a diagnosis of osteoporosis. Regular bone scans are carried out to monitor this important area of health. So, the physical effects roll on!

*

OLIVIA ANTHONY
Olivia is a 44-year-old living
with anorexia nervosa and bulimia

My poor body has been through so much. I really should love my body and thank it for not giving up on me. I've treated it horribly, and yet it has kept me alive. My eating disorder started when I was thirteen. I didn't suffer a lot of physical symptoms until college. That's when ED really took over and I suffered more. I was cold all the time. I had swollen glands in my face and had acid reflux. I covered my teeth with foil before purging, but after a while I didn't care enough to do even that.

Later, in my late twenties and early thirties, I fainted a lot. My son was little and would run over to me, telling me to wake up. That was awful. I had a bruise at the base of my spine that was always sore because I had lost all my fat. I lost hair, and I had a seizure. I tore my throat from purging, so my throat bled.

When I was forty I relapsed again. I journaled throughout, and decided to include several posts here that can better show how I was affected by my marriage to ED. My journal was a private blog for my therapist to read before sessions.

January: *I had xxx calories today and then did two workouts, the Butt Bible Upper and Lower. I then cleaned the bathrooms, tubs and all. I'm getting faster at catching myself before I pass out. But it was quite annoying, as I was cleaning, to constantly be getting lightheaded and not be able to see. I worried I was going to fall into the tub and break teeth. That would not be cool. I woke up every single hour last night, all night long. I had cramps and pain from irritable bowel syndrome, but didn't have diarrhea. I wonder if I have ketoacidosis. I wake up all night with a dry mouth, having to pee, and in the morning my room always smells weird. I have to air it out for fifteen minutes. I know I brought this on myself. But I can't help but worry; it's a sucky cycle to be in. A few days ago both of my kidneys hurt in the morning. And last night I woke up all night with my right kidney hurting. It still hurts. I made an eye appointment for Friday. For a week my left eye has been blurry and irritated. I thought it'd go away because I assumed it was from purging. I burst a couple of blood vessels, and it was irritated right after that. So, I'll find out Friday. I'm not telling him about the purging. And I am wondering about asking Dr. R about taking xxx to help with sleeping. I can't sleep. I'm so effing sick of it. And I know that eating better would help, but it's not that easy.* 01/31/12

I know it's Ed's fault for not sleeping much last night. I can't make myself eat enough. I'm so mad! I was all shaky this morning, and my heart hurt. Dammit. Oh, well, what can I do? You would think that my heart hurting, kidneys hurting, my waking up all night, low energy, etc., would be enough to make me eat. One would think so. But I can't! And then I worry that something is wrong with my body because I'm not dropping the weight like I was, and I'm still undereating for someone my height. Wouldn't one still lose weight at xxx calories per day? So of course there is no way that I'll feel safe eating xxx, much less xxx or, god forbid xxx calories/day. I would gain weight for sure. 01/31/12

February: *Just a quickie before going to the eye doc. Why does my body wake up all night, having to pee? And it's not a lot of pee, just a little. I've never had this before with the ED. Why does it happen? Maybe because I'm older and my uterus is pushing on my bladder! I went to bed with a massive headache, and couldn't take any pills because of an empty stomach. When I got up at night, I still had it, and I had it when I got up. I ate some yogurt with banana when I got up, so I took some ibuprofen and it's just now finally going away. Anyway, still nothing on the period. It completely ended Tuesday night. Two-day period. Okay, going to the eye doc. I'm sorry I'm such a boring, obsessive patient.* 02/3/12

Oh, my god. I thought I was going to die. Seriously, I just binged on xxx, ate them xxx minutes ago. Went in to purge after xxx minutes. They lumped in my throat! I had to pound my esophagus. Now I'm scared to death. I still want to purge, but I'm so worried. Each xxx is xxx calories! I don't know what I'm going to do. 02/11/12 11:54 p.m.

121

Have been lightheaded all day; couldn't see, mouth was numb. Then worked out and it happened during the workout. And then for the last twenty minutes of my workout I had a lovely ocular migraine. They're not painful, but they block your vision; a shimmering moon was in the entire left side of my vision. I've been getting those since fall. I called the clinic the first time I got one, maybe September or October, and they didn't tell me what it was, just that it wasn't serious. They always last between thirty to forty minutes. More annoying than anything, except that they usually precipitate a migraine. At least for me. I don't know about others. So I have that to look forward to. 02/11/12

So, as much as I am scared of dying from purging, I drank another glass of warm water, swished it around inside me, and went back to purge. I purged it all up—all of it. And then took my bath and cried. I can't stop! I feel like a drug addict who can't stop on her own. I can't stop! I know it's killing me. I know it's killing my son's mother, and that isn't enough to make me stop! It should be! I'm so sad. I don't care what the side effects are from the meds anymore. I think the side effects would be better than dying and suffering from ED! I can't take it anymore. I am crying right now and am so sick of this. I have been down this very familiar path before and it is impossible to stop without help. Please, I beg of you, please don't give up on me. I know and I have been told how much of a difficult case I am. I know that and I apologize. I just cannot do it on my own. God, I want to just bawl! 02/12/2012 12:16 a.m.

I just took a shower and felt sick. I took my pulse for a minute, and it's xxx. Is that because I have only had xxx calories, and it's almost 6 p.m.? What is causing that? Dammit. I didn't want to eat today. I googled to see what's causing that; all I saw was something about diabetes and hypoglycemia, so I bet it is blood sugar. 02/19/12 05:47 p.m.

I wasn't going to eat today. I had coffee with half-n-half and that's it. But with my heart rate so fast, I figured it was low blood sugar. I was trying to read the instructions for making dinner, and I had to say the words out loud and was so confused, and had to reread it over and over. I was scared! My hands were jittery and I just felt wrong. So I sat down and ate xxx. I feel better, and my heartrate now is xxx. My hands are still really jittery, but that could be the medication, although I haven't had the shaky hands since Thursday. I think the initial shaky hands was my brain maybe just being on the medication? Is that possible? Who freaking knows. My body has a mind of its own. I had to make cocoa. Still felt off. I had xxx of cocoa, so I'm mad I had xxx now. 02/19/12 06:09 p.m.

I have that low blood sugar again. I'm so scared. I've got sweaty hands, and my teeth are chattering. I took a hot bath and was cold. My heart is racing and my hands are shaking. I am covered in two blankets! So I'm making another xxx of hot chocolate. I called the clinic and left a message to see if she can fit me in tomorrow anyway. I am scaring myself. I know I can never skip breakfast again. I just thought I could fast today since I had xxx yesterday. I'm wrong. I'm freaking out with this low blood sugar thing. As I was running the bath, I was peeing (in the toilet, not the tub!) and drank a full xxx-ounce tumbler. I don't want to add dehydration on top of it. I'm scared. But as I was sitting there, I told myself that all the tests that Dr. R did showed that I'm fine. So part of me thought that I was just being worried for nothing. But my heart was pounding so fast, and I was shaking from being cold, my teeth were chattering, my hands are sweaty, and I got so scared since it's the second time today that's happened. I wasn't lightheaded even once today, though. So that's good. I just worry about leaving Liam. As I was sitting on the toilet, I was thinking about how I'm just so tired of fighting this. I fantasized briefly about dying from this to make it end. But then I immediately thought of my son and how I cannot let myself give up. That's when I got in the tub and thought about calling the clinic. I just want to hurry up and get that intake appointment over with, and see about seeing a nutritionist and getting my head screwed on tight. Do you think I will get extra sessions with you? I don't want to get my hopes up. I haven't figured out yet what I'm going to have to tell Liam about everything. Even a nutritionist... maybe just that I want us to eat healthier. I don't really care about that right now. I'll figure it out.

Update: Heartrate is down to xxx now after the cocoa. I feel better. Dammit. I don't ever, ever want this again. I have never had so many problems with symptoms before with ED than I'm having now. My body is conspiring against me. I really can't believe how many symptoms I've had this time around. My body is probably pissed off and complaining at me. I mean, when I got down to xxx, I was fainting out cold, but that was all. I am in a "healthy weight range" for almost five feet ten inches, yet am having so many symptoms. It's scary! 02/19/12 11:01 p.m.

I'm really hoping that by eating, it will keep hypoglycemia away. Those symptoms sucked so bad. It was like the flu, when you're shaking and sweating, only your heart is also pounding and racing and you just feel sick. I don't ever want to experience that again. So I ate. And I hope that I can keep that away today. I really feel like I keep complaining all the time about all the things that keep happening to my body. But, it's all scary to me! Unfortunately, being scared over and over can't scare ED out of me. That's the sad part. 02/20/12

My toes are tingling in both feet. I'm so relieved I'll be seeing Dr. R tomorrow morning. I'm really worried about these symptoms. And I wasn't going to say anything about it, but both my kidneys have been sore since I got up. I thought it'd go away. I've been drinking a ton of water. I'm so damn pissed off; I'm going to have to learn to kick ED to the curb. I just want to cry, thinking about losing him. F***ed up, I know. But I know I need to learn to live without him. 02/23/12

I went to bed at 12:30 a.m. last night, but couldn't fall asleep. Then at 1 a.m. my left foot was numb! I couldn't fall asleep after that because of that numb foot! I am so worried. I last looked at the clock around 3:30 a.m. So I fell asleep around then. And then woke up at 5 a.m. The sheets were soaked. My hair was soaked, my face, my shirt, my shorts. I drank some water, peed a lot, then went back to bed. I fell asleep until 8:17 a.m.

Again, the sheets were wet, my hair and face were soaked, as well as my T-shirt. And then, my torso felt like it was vibrating. My hands were shaking. So I got up. I ate xxx at 8:35 a.m. My heart rate was xxx! Am I doing permanent damage here? I am going to have to write notes for my appointment with Dr. R tomorrow, because I know I won't remember the details about everything.

March: I couldn't sleep at all last night. I know it's because I have been eating xxx calories the last two days in a row. I woke up sweaty and with a headache. My body can't take it. Seriously. I'm not kidding. I used to be able to be with ED for years and years in a row, and I didn't have these symptoms. I admit that during the bad bulimic years it was a different kind of torture, but with restricting it was different. Now that I think about it, maybe it has to do with the fact that I was overweight first this time. Maybe that's why? I'm not a scientist, so I have no idea. I just know that my body is not happy that I'm doing this all over again. 03/01/12

Face plant. It was bound to happen. I woke up at 6:15 a.m. and went into the bathroom to pee. Before I knew it, I fainted and fell on my face. Completely on my face. The noise woke Liam up. I have a rug burn on my chin, it's swollen, and my right wrist hit the wooden garbage can, so I have a scrape there too. Thank goodness I at least fell on the padded bathmat and not the linoleum. I'm so glad. I kept waking up after that, and I was getting the shakes. I feel better after eating. 03/05/12

Lovely. I just put on my face. I have a lump on my left eyebrow. It's sore from the face plant. Lovely. I'm just so classy—fainting because I'm starving myself. Proud day for me. 03/05/12

I miss sleep! I took my two xxx tabs at 1:15 a.m. and couldn't fall asleep. My mind wouldn't stop thinking about everything. Plus, my feet were tingling, so I worried about that. I slept almost two hours, woke at almost 5 a.m. I was wide awake, so I took two more xxx tabs. I slept till about 8 a.m. Then my brain was doing that weird thing; all I can describe it as is a slight vibration. It feels like my brain is humming a little. My heart was doing that too. So I worried about blood sugar issues and got up, slowly, and had a banana. I slept for another hour after that. Then my brain and heart did that vibration thing again. So I just got up and had xxx! I've had xxx already and it's 10:30 a.m. But my brain and heart quit doing that humming vibration thing. And part of my not being able to sleep is because my chin hurts. I sleep on my stomach and I know I must have tweaked the vertebrae in my neck when I fell on my face at that angle, because my neck feels like it needs an alignment. So I had my regular sleep issues going on, plus my body was sore from my face plant. And then I kept waking up because my right hipbone hurt. I bruised that too! No wonder I woke Liam. He can sleep through the smoke alarms! I fell so hard and fast. I miss sleep! And I'm aiming for xxx! Yes. It's been a while since I've done the xxx-calorie plan. It triggered my purging last time I tried that. But, fainting is not on my list of accomplishments, and eating xxx calories a day might help. It's a start! 03/06/2012 10:38 a.m.

April: *I am so sick of myself. Of ED. Why does it feel so good, and bad, to purge? It feels good when it forcefully comes up, but then I feel like a loser. I thought of that last time I purged. I was having a hard time getting it up, and thought, god, I'm not even a man, and I'm having a hard time getting it up. Ha. Kinda funny, though.* 04/11/12

I wish so much that there was a med for ED. I mean, people with other mental illnesses find such relief with meds. But with ED, there is no magic pill to take away the constant nagging and pestering and bullying. God, I'm so pissed. Why do I have to be so gullible and fall into ED's arms so easily? It's like a battered wife. I know ED's not good for me. I know ED's abusive and could kill me. Yet I love ED and get comfort from ED and am not totally alone with ED. I need a restraining order. I need a hit man. I need someone to take ED out! 04/16/12 6 a.m.

I am just so mad at myself. I can't stop. This is going to be the death of me. I know that I can't keep doing this for another twenty years, or even ten, or one. It sucks that this coping mechanism could kill me. I'm so mad, and I just want to cry. I don't want to see my dad at all this summer. And I know I'd feel like I had to pretend around my siblings and Mom. I'd feel like I have to pretend that nothing happened. And I just can't do that. I don't care anymore about hurting people's feelings by not going. I'll be too stressed out, and I just don't want to deal with all that. I just want to cry. 04/22/12 10:28 p.m.

I'm mad at myself for purging and feeling so out of control when this is supposed to make me feel in control. I'm sick of worrying about being caught by Liam. I'm sick of smelling like vomit. I'm sick of worrying about stupid health issues. I'm sick of not knowing who I really am and what I want to do with myself. I'm scared. And I'm sick of being scared. I'm sick of worrying about the worst that can happen. I know that most likely I won't be raped again, or abused. But I can't help myself. I'm so tired of living. 04/22/2012 11:42 p.m.

I'm hungry. I hope and pray that I can stop myself from freaking out and purging. Just seriously, kill me now. It'd be easier to croak than to fight this. I'm forty, and I'm purging like a sixteen-year-old girl. I am sick of feeling like a loser. 04/24/2012

*

CHRISTINE BASTONE
Christine is a 49-year-old living
with binge eating disorder

I'm sure that my weight affects my health. I'm sure that my lack of physical exercise affects it as well. I have tried both to lose weight and to exercise on a regular basis. I have even succeeded at both for short periods of time. One day I came across Paul McKenna on TV. I loved his approach—it's so simple and yet so powerful: eat when you're hungry, eat what you want (no food is off limits), eat slowly, and stop when you think you might be full. Unfortunately, the only part of those things that I'm good at is eating what I want. I don't like to wait until I'm hungry. I have way more emotional hunger than physical hunger. I also eat too fast, and don't want to stop until I'm really full. For a while there, though, I did do all those things, especially eat slower. And I did lose some weight.

Because of my chronic fatigue, which makes me feel like I've been hit by a truck when I exercise, I had absolutely no luck until I found the Wii dance games. We bought them all and for a few months I did some every day. It was absolutely wonderful, because doing them didn't bring on my symptoms, and for the first time in a very long time I occasionally felt the rush of endorphins instead. I'm not sure why I stopped. I probably got really busy and had to temporarily drop it from my schedule, got out of the habit, and the temporary break turned out to be much longer than I had planned. But those two things are the only success I have had in trying to lose weight, get in better shape, and minimize the physical damage of my eating disorder.

*

LISA BRUNS
Lisa is a 52-year-old living
with binge eating disorder

My eating disorder has affected my health. I have osteoarthritis and have hip and back issues. After having gastric bypass, I lost one hundred pounds but have gained thirty back. It's been a struggle. I had back surgery and can't seem to bounce back. Lack of exercise because of back issues hasn't helped. I don't know if I can lose the weight.

*

LYNDA CHELDELIN FELL
Lynda is a 50-year-old living
with binge eating disorder

At my heaviest, my knees hurt and activities I loved were becoming harder to do. I've always enjoyed gardening. Digging in fresh dirt was always a joy for me; it was how I recharged my battery. I loved listening to the kids chatter as I tended to this plant or that flower. I loved the sight of a seedling emerging from the rich, moist soil or a flower in full bloom. But weighing over two hundred pounds was hard on my frame. My joints were starting to break down, and I knew that comorbidities such as diabetes and high blood pressure weren't far off in my future. My body was beginning to pay the price for years of bingeing. This was part of my catalyst for change.

Ten years later, after shedding one hundred pounds and finally fit and healthy, I still have joint problems. I also have excessive skin on my arms, legs, and belly. I'm aware that surgery can remove the excess skin, but it also keeps me honest. It's my reminder of what happens when I don't treat my body kindly by keeping my eating disorder in check. Clothing hides the extra skin easily enough, and I've managed to avoid diabetes and high blood pressure. I definitely wasn't in denial about the damage I was doing to myself. In fact, it scared me. I spent a number of years in the medical field, and was well aware I was playing with fire. But the powerful cravings overrode the looming threat of consequence. Nonetheless, damage done doesn't magically evaporate when one loses weight. It's for life.

*

JUSTINE HILDEN
Justine is a 27-year-old living
with binge eating disorder

I struggle with binge eating and compulsive overeating. I have gained a significant amount of weight, nearly doubled my weight. It's been eight years, and I have been lucky in many ways; no diabetes or high blood pressure. However, I do struggle with sleep apnea, knee pain, and plantar fasciitis. Things that used to be easy for me are no longer as easy. Physical activity became very difficult. Walking was harder, breathing became more labored, and I was sore. I had enjoyed doing physical activity prior to my eating disorder. I loved to hike, bike, and walk. For so many years, they were things I avoided like the plague, because if I did those activities, and I struggled, that would only be confirming and reminding me of my struggles with weight and my eating disorder, which I often tried to ignore and pretend it wasn't my reality. It has taken many years, support from my family, and support from my eating disorder team. I am not working out in a healthy way. Weight loss is what I want, of course, but right now I am focusing on being active. I now do kickboxing and strength training regularly, and have completed 5K, 7K and even a 10K. I am still able to do that at my current weight. I am able to see what my body can do. Even though I am far from my ideal weight, my body is doing things I didn't think I could do, or things I was afraid to do. I had let my weight and my eating disorder stop me from trying to do the things I once loved and enjoyed.

*

LYDIA KENYON
Lydia is a 22-year-old living
with anorexia nervosa

I had extremely low blood pressure when I went to the doctor for the first time when I began recovery. I also had some lanugo on my face. The doctor suspects I have osteopenia, but I haven't been tested for that yet. I think my body is naturally used to being thin (no one in my family is very heavy), so I think that was a blessing in disguise during my illness. I'm sure my body is damaged in ways I cannot see, but I have been very lucky.

*

REBEKKAH KOONS
Rebekkah is a 29-year-old living with
an eating disorder not otherwise specified

I don't know if it's directly related to my past eating disorder, but during that time I had such bad anxiety, that my heart would jump all over the place and my blood pressure would rise to dangerous levels. I've been on blood pressure medicine every day since I turned twenty-four. Also, I've had lab work many times to check my electrolytes, and continue to have routine blood work.

*

MONICA MIRKES
Monica is a 58-year-old living
with binge eating disorder

The extra weight I put on really impacted my knees. I was diagnosed with arthritis. I couldn't believe I was having trouble going up and down stairs.

*

RUTH PAPALAS
Ruth is a 58-year-old living
with binge eating disorder

At first I just thought it was uncomfortable and I needed to go on yet another diet. My feet, legs and back hurt. I got pregnant and ended up with toxemia (preeclampsia) twice. The first time, they never told me I had it until after I had my son and was at my six-week follow-up. Six years later, the second pregnancy resulted in an emergency C-section and a premature two-pound eight-ounce baby. I never lost much weight after the first baby, and certainly not after the second baby. I was not aware of what caused toxemia. Much later I learned that diet and obesity are two causes of toxemia.

Two of my biggest health fears are heart attack and diabetes. This is mostly because my dad died at sixty-two years old from a heart attack and both of my grandmothers had diabetes.

My first clue that I was seriously damaging myself physically was when I started coughing after walking even short distances. Someone anonymously slipped a brochure about asthma on my desk. I read it and sought out my family doctor. He sent me to a lung specialist (pulmonologist) who diagnosed me with asthma. The doctor asked if any of my immediate family had died of a heart attack. I said, "Yes, my dad." He said most people don't realize how closely the lungs and the heart are related, and if you have lung issues you may then end up with heart issues.

I had been to several doctors, including my family doctor and diet doctors looking for a magic pill or cure—anything. One day while reading *Women's World Magazine*, I read an article about gastric bypass. I studied up on the surgery. I read books, articles, and checked the internet. I checked online. I made an appointment. My family was not really supportive. In fact, my husband told me that if I lived through it, he would consider it. He had a gastric bypass a year later.

*

DEBBIE PFIFFNER
Debbie is a 56-year-old living
with anorexia nervosa

First and foremost, I have severe osteoporosis and have had it for many years. There are certain things I am unable to do, like skiing, horseback riding, ice skating, or participating in any type of activity where there is a chance of falling and breaking a bone. As of my last bone density test, my hipbones are affected the most, and even a small fall could result in a fracture. That type of fracture could actually kill me. Living in Minnesota, land of ten thousand patches of ice on sidewalks and parking lots, sometimes just walking is dangerous.

I also went through menopause at the age of forty. Although they cannot definitively prove that my eating disorder caused the menopause, they can't rule it out. Another health issue I have is small fiber neuropathy in my legs. It can be extremely painful and uncomfortable. Although the neuropathy is not a direct result of my eating disorder, but rather a direct result of the many years I spent as an active alcoholic, my low body fat is a predominant factor in the amount of pain I experience.

*

DENISE PURCELL
Denise is a 50-year-old living
with anorexia nervosa and bulimia

My food disorders have affected me in some areas. I had an ulcer and acid reflux because of making myself throw up. I have had digestive problems ranging from constipation to spastic colon. My teeth are not the strongest. I do have low blood pressure, but didn't realize it until I had surgeries on my back and was hospitalized longer because they couldn't stabilize me.

*

HADDI TREBISOVSKY
Haddi is a 29-year-old living
with anorexia nervosa

My eating disorder never became severe enough to affect my health in any lasting way, which I am so grateful for. However, I did frequently get migraines from skipping meals. Migraines have long plagued me, and only recently have they become manageable after I cut dairy out of my diet, but that's an entirely different story! I know that the low blood sugar I experienced from restricting was a major trigger in making me lightheaded and giving me headaches and migraines, along with very tense muscles. At the time, I wasn't fully conscious of the effect my decision was having on my health, but after a while I started to make the connection, and begrudgingly ate a snack if I felt pain coming on.

*

CHAPTER NINE

Dominating Our Lives

> Many of our choices are between good and evil. The choices we make, however, determine to a large extent our happiness or our unhappiness, because we have to live with the consequences of our choices. -JAMES E. FAUST

While eating disorders often lead to serious and sometimes life-threatening physical consequences, they also affect other areas of our lives. Dominating our thoughts and minds, the intrusion impacts our careers, relationships, and even our mental stability. How has your eating disorder affected other areas of your life?

*

JUNE ALEXANDER
June is a 65-year-old living
beyond anorexia nervosa

The physical consequences of my eating disorder have had far-reaching effects on my emotions. Especially in my early years, indeed until my late forties, I was in denial that health issues were connected to my eating disorder. Equally important was the lack of information and education available to help make me aware of the risks and consequences, and provide support in acquiring skills to develop self-loving rather than self-harming behaviors and thought patterns.

I mentioned some emotional effects in an earlier response, and will elaborate further here. Often one thing led to another. For instance, at some level I knew I could not go on having baby after baby in a bid to control my eating disorder. But I could not articulate the fear or shame of reasons why I wanted to keep having babies. I knew I had to have a tubal ligation before returning home with my fourth baby in four years. Otherwise I would become focused on a fifth pregnancy. A tubal ligation would prevent my use of pregnancy as a lever to fight my thoughts, and while I knew that financially we could not afford a fifth baby—I needed to work to help support our family—the thought of losing a path for attempted self-management worried me. My gynecologist said, "I would prefer you to be thirty before operating, but because you have four children I'll do it now." He preferred to wait eight weeks after the birth to allow my uterus to contract. But if I went home without the operation, I knew my thoughts would rage and I would want a fifth baby. Rather than tell the doctor this, I said I'd have difficulty organizing childcare to be able to return to the hospital in eight weeks. The operation was scheduled six days after my fourth baby's birth, the day after my twenty-sixth birthday.

Descent into chronic anxiety and depression was swift. Within two years I was suicidal. I was exhausted from fighting my eating disorder. I hated it and hated myself. I couldn't get away from it. I could see no way out. It was at this time, driven by love for my children, that I shared my long-held eating disorder secret with a doctor for the first time. I feared I would be packed off to a mental asylum and lose custody of my children. Instead, the doctor told me I had a chemical problem. He said some pills would help fix it. Six years of misdiagnosis followed.

In my early thirties, with my marriage falling apart and now, for the first time, under the care of a psychiatrist who saw me beyond the layers of illness, I also sought spiritual counseling. I met with the local church minister, who had gained my trust, to discuss my feelings. I'd always been moral-minded, but now, with my marriage in tatters (my eating disorder had convinced me that another man held the key to freedom from its torment), my values were flying out the window.

During a three-hour session in which I emptied a tissue box, I poured out my guilt. I described how I had used the terms of my pregnancies to try to gain control over my tormentor. I feared I'd had my children for the wrong reasons. The kindly minister said there was no right or wrong reason to have a child. "Each one is special," he said, helping to ease my guilt and shame, and put my mind at rest. "You love your children, and this is most important." After listening to me unravel the complexity of my life, he gently suggested that I might find committing fully to God as the safest option for healing my soul. But while I loved God for being so patient with me, I couldn't contemplate that thought. My thinking process at that time was totally inflexible. Dominated by the eating disorder, it was black and white. All or nothing. To contemplate anything in between was too scary. Way too scary. My anxiety was extreme. My hold on reality was exceedingly fragile.

In considering how the eating disorder has affected my overall health, I feel a sense of grief that this illness developed in my brain in childhood and proceeded to make me its prisoner for the next four decades. The detrimental effect on relationships, as well as health, was immense. I feel a sense of loss, for my childhood was cut short. And the eating disorder bully influenced adolescence and early adulthood in multiple, negative ways. The burden of secrets loaded with shame, guilt, anxiety and self-loathing were, at times, debilitating. Death often loomed as the only way out. So, there is sadness. But there is also relief, in relation to the revelation in my forties that some of the physical consequences of my illness could be attended to, and their effects ameliorated if not reversed.

By attending to the physical consequences of my illness, with love and self-care directed by my treatment team, I became aware that slowly, tiny step by tiny step, I was restoring my authentic self. While there was life, there was hope.

*

OLIVIA ANTHONY
Olivia is a 44-year-old living
with anorexia nervosa and bulimia

I vacillate between feeling worried that I've done long-term damage to my body, perhaps taking years off of my life, to knowing that I chose, in a pre-birth soul plan, to have ED as my challenge in this life, so it was meant to be. I still have sadness whenever I think about how I worried my loved ones, especially my son. And I really do have sadness for my body, too. I did so much abuse to my body. It was really tough rereading my journal when putting things together for this book. It took me back to the awful, desperate feelings I was experiencing. I also feel amazed and proud of myself for coming through ED! I am strong! Sure, I nearly gave up and nearly killed myself with ED as my lover, but I am here! And that makes me proud. ED is a fierce enemy. But I am alive!

*

CHRISTINE BASTONE
Christine is a 49-year-old living
with binge eating disorder

I don't dwell on the physical consequences of my eating disorder with regard to my health. That may change as I get older, but right now I focus on the physical consequences of what my eating disorder does to my appearance.

*

LISA BRUNS
Lisa is a 52-year-old living
with binge eating disorder

I shut down. I stay in the house. I don't want to be around family or friends. I don't want anyone to see me. I was a diabetic, had high blood pressure, and needed a double hip replacement and back surgery before gastric. I'm terrified that I'll get the diabetes back and the weight gain will cause further problems with my back.

*

LYNDA CHELDELIN FELL
Lynda is a 50-year-old living
with binge eating disorder

I was thin and fit when I first met my husband. My pendulum was at the extreme edge—I was exercising three hours a day. I fell head over heels in love with Mr. Right; he was a good man. And a good man deserved the truth. I needed to tell him that I had a problem with food. But how could I describe something I didn't understand? I wasn't sure how to confess, but I felt strongly that he deserved to know so he could judge for himself whether my problem was a deal breaker. It wasn't. At the time, I was thin and tan. My current physical appearance belied the ugly truth.

We married within nine months of meeting, and two months later I was pregnant. My strict eating habits swung to the other side of the pendulum, and down the rabbit hole I went. When our daughter was ten months old I became pregnant again. I hadn't shed the weight from my prior pregnancy, and gained even more with this pregnancy. Being pregnant afforded two bonuses: eating for two, and maternity clothes came with elastic waistbands.

After the birth of my fourth child, I was clinically obese. I worried whether my husband still found me desirable. The frequency of our intimacy wasn't affected, but my large size inhibited my sexual freedom. And that bothered my husband. He liked to see me naked, but my shame trumped. Lights remained off, and body exposure was limited. Experimenting with oils and other sensual items were now out of the question. I knew my husband loved me, and he never gave me reason to feel ashamed. Yet I remained worried. According to movies and magazines, thin women are highly prized trophies. I knew how I stacked up against them. Literally. I did whatever it took to camouflage my growing obesity. And I continued to question how my husband could love me when I hated myself for being so weak.

The relationship that suffered most was with my in-laws. My husband was born and raised in Australia. My husband's mother spent life in a boarding school. Her judgment of Americans was swift and harsh: we are loud, rogue rednecks. Having an American daughter-in-law was nothing to be proud of.

In 2007, we went to Australia for a five-week visit. I was one year in to my food sobriety, and still on thin ice. Although I yearned to try Aussie meat pies, sausage rolls, Lamingtons and pavlova, I stuck to my eating routine like superglue. My mother-in-law didn't take kindly to my strict eating habits, and was greatly offended when I declined a serving of her carefully crafted trifle. To do so meant very poor manners on my part. Secretly, I drooled over her confection but was too embarrassed to admit I had an eating disorder. I doubted she would understand how one small taste could swing my pendulum toward defeat, so it wasn't a dialogue I wanted to open. Offended at how little I ate, my mother-in-law's distaste for me grew with each passing meal. I did the best I could while visiting Australia. I helped with chores, did dishes, our children were well mannered, and I made sure we were easy guests. But no matter how hard I tried to earn my mother-in-law's approval, my eating disorder habits were too great of an offense.

*

JUSTINE HILDEN
Justine is a 27-year-old living
with binge eating disorder

I have my up and down days when it comes to how I feel about myself, my weight, and the physical consequences of my eating disorder. There are days when I feel very disappointed in myself that I would let myself nearly double my weight. It's the perfectionist in me. There are days when I feel as if I am near recovery. It really depends on the day. I have not been in denial that my health issues are connected to my eating disorder. I have always been very aware. I just get frustrated that I don't just lose weight (as if it were an easy process). I blame myself for letting my weight get to this point, for getting to this place where my health and physical well-being are impacted. I have really had to practice patience and compassion for myself. I try to take it day by day and seek support when I am struggling with those ups and downs.

*

LYDIA KENYON
Lydia is a 22-year-old living
with anorexia nervosa

It makes me sad that I was hurting myself so much, and yet it didn't matter to me. I was so scared that one day when I was exercising I would suffer a heart attack—but that didn't stop me from exercising and eating very little. It makes me very upset to look back on my past. I know I hurt a lot of people by saying things that hurt them, or not saying things when they needed me to. Anorexia made me very selfish, and I am ashamed of that.

*

REBEKKAH KOONS
Rebekkah is a 29-year-old living with
an eating disorder not otherwise specified

I take medicine at night just to turn my thoughts off. It also helps when I'm having anxiety over gaining too much weight. I do take medicine that cuts my appetite, but from a medical standpoint I need it to be able to concentrate on work and coaching.

*

MONICA MIRKES
Monica is a 58-year-old living
with binge eating disorder

Depressed, discouraged, hopeless. I feel like saying what's the point? Nothing I did made a difference, like counting calories or watching what I ate. If only I could have had some weight loss, I would at least have been encouraged to continue.

*

RUTH PAPALAS
Ruth is a 58-year-old living
with binge eating disorder

I come across to most people as a fairly confident person. People don't know that I try on four to five different combinations of clothing every day to see if I can somehow hide this or that bulge. I have found myself in denial many times that my health issues were connected to my ED. I've had myself tested for thyroid, diabetes, and a couple of other things, just *knowing* that if I were diagnosed with a disease or a disorder of some kind I would receive a magic prescription—and I would be cured. It can't just be that I eat too much. It can't be! I am finally honest with myself. It's me. I have issues. I stress about everything. I worry about my kids, my mom and siblings, finances, the government, the future in general. What will happen to me if something happens to my husband? What will happen to him if something happens to me? I'm a giant ball of emotional stress! In the meantime, I always feel self-conscious about how I look to other people. Yep—a giant emotional stress ball! That's me!

*

DEBBIE PFIFFNER
Debbie is a 56-year-old living
with anorexia nervosa

I just had an incident come up this past week. My husband and I drove past the community center by our house, where there is an outdoor skating rink. I loved to ice skate. I have not skated in years. I am also very, very bad at it, but it never stopped me from loving it. I told my husband that if there was one thing in this world I would like to do more than anything, it would be to put on my skates and go skating on that little ice rink. Later on I ended up in tears, crying over how much I have lost due to my eating disorder. I was angry, I was grief-stricken, I was blaming myself for letting all this happen. The strongest emotion I feel is definitely anger at myself for letting this happen. Whether I actually "let" this happen is irrelevant to me. I still blame myself, and spend time wishing I could go back and do something to prevent it from happening.

*

DENISE PURCELL
Denise is a 50-year-old living
with anorexia nervosa and bulimia

I am well aware of just about everything it can do to me. I am a
very good researcher when it comes to things. It didn't change much
in what I did. I just knew I could develop problems; maybe not now,
but later on in life. I don't like to feel emotions of any kind very much.
My thinking when I was dealing with the anorexia was that if I could
just be small enough, then maybe I could just disappear.

*

HADDI TREBISOVSKY
Haddi is a 29-year-old living
with anorexia nervosa

I wasn't in denial that my health was affected. I truly just wasn't
able to make the connection when I was young. Migraines, however,
really took an emotional toll on me. Many times I felt it would be
better if I were dead than to be suffering the way I was. At my worst,
I was getting headaches at least five times a week, with a migraine
typically once or more a week.

*

Hope is the only bee that
makes honey without flowers.
ROBERT GREEN INGERSOLL

*

CHAPTER TEN

Hiding From Family

To effectively communicate, we must realize that we are all different in the way we perceive the world and use this understanding as a guide to our communication with others. -TONY ROBBINS

People living with eating disorders become masters at hiding secrets. Protecting our precarious behavior at all costs, we become secretive, clever, and clandestine. Yet complications with our physical health sometimes threaten to reveal the truth. Did family, friends, or your doctor correlate an eating disorder with some of your health issues?

*

JUNE ALEXANDER
June is a 65-year-old living
beyond anorexia nervosa

Until my late forties I lacked the skills to know when a thought could be attributed to the true me, or belonged to the eating disorder, or was influenced by prescription drugs. Finding a way out of the dark forest of the eating disorder was difficult, but slowly another thread of self was found, and another, and another. By weaving them together, I began to rebuild *me*. I was in my mid-forties when a dietitian, aware of the latest research in the eating disorder field, in family-based treatment, and also in mindfulness, managed to gain my trust. I began to see that I had to learn to trust myself, and not the eating disorder, before I could have a healthy relationship with others or myself. She explained that the eating disorder thoughts were not of the true me. This insight was a great comfort and relief.

Sorting the illness thoughts from true thoughts was a big job, and it followed that I then needed to catch the illness thoughts and defuse them before they took off. This task, commenced at age forty-seven, of getting in touch with my feelings, and taking care of them, would take eight years to accomplish. At the same time, I would succeed in my long-held challenge of eating three meals and three snacks a day. This sounds like a simple feat, but after thirty years of food ruling my life, it was remarkable. My diary became a place for recording progress and practicing self-awareness.

As noted in chapter eight, two operations assisted my recovery of self: a hysterectomy and the titanium rod in my cervical spine. My neurosurgeon, besides caring about my spine, cared about me. He arranged for a psychiatry colleague to visit my bedside. I was told that an internal saboteur was causing constant chaos in both my inner and outer life. To be free, I had to identify and eliminate it. This fresh insight helped me to externalize the anorexia and view it as separate from self.

As a step toward building self-belief, the neurosurgeon and psychiatrist insisted I repeat the mantra: "I deserve to be treated with respect," over and over until it became a reality in my brain. It is tough, awfully tough, getting out of the anorexia prison with your life but without your childhood family. Unfortunately, my family of origin had developed a way of life that did not include me by the time I emerged from my eating disorder. I cope by counting blessings. Things provided in childhood have helped me get through—a love of writing, a love of nature, and the love of my grandma who wrote on a scrap of paper, "This is June's." I'm sure my parents loved me, but they didn't know how to cope. I had to change, to live, but they had become comfortable in their groove. So I did not feel my family of origin were supportive of my secondary health issues.

My family of origin was able to appreciate and recognize the physical health issues, for these were seen as acceptable and real, but were unable to understand the connection with my mental health. Mental illness was considered a personal weakness; it was simply a matter of pulling your socks up, "Stop thinking about yourself so much," and getting on with life. While the lack of understanding and support from my family of origin definitely impeded and slowed my recovery, I feel fortunate to have met others who've been supportive. I owe my life to a network of support that includes my children's dad, my children and grandchildren, friends, psychiatrist, therapists, doctors, neurosurgeon, minister of religion, and faith in God.

I lost my family of origin, and my marriage, but have gained another family in recovery—a family comprising people from all walks of life in the eating disorder field. This family of choice nurtures my fledgling self-belief. Respecting the person beyond the illness makes a world of difference. Respect gives hope. Today, my eating disorder has been replaced with the joy and love of family, self and life.

Writing has enabled the re-storying of hurtful, traumatic experiences in a way that allows me to embrace the current moment. The passion for writing that helped me to survive privately has become a sword in fighting eating disorders around the world, by disseminating evidence-based research. Love, faith, and three nutritious meals and three snacks a day, together with walks by the seashore, are my maintenance program.

I'll never know if I am the person I would have been if I had not developed anorexia nervosa at age eleven. What I do know is that I am now free of the eating disorder bully. Its effects linger, however. Anxiety and stress no longer manifest in food behaviors and thoughts, but instead find outlets in physical symptoms which puzzle neurosurgeons, neurologists and psychiatrists alike. For instance, bouts of severe neurological pain, chronic urticaria and loss of mobility in the upper spine have been found to have no physical explanation.

The challenge is to self-love and self-care at all times and to promptly attend to and achieve a resolution for every issue, no matter how minor it may seem. Thyroid levels, blood counts and blood pressure are all regularly checked. My experience has shown that body and self are intrinsically entwined, and that care must embody the two for good health and happiness to ensue.

THROUGH THE EYES OF AN EATING DISORDER

*

OLIVIA ANTHONY
Olivia is a 44-year-old living
with anorexia nervosa and bulimia

Oh, yes. All but one psychiatrist, who does not specialize in eating disorders, told me many times how ED was to blame for all the numerous problems I was having, physically and mentally. My doctors and therapists definitely knew my ED was doing a lot of damage. My friends also understood exactly what was going on. That was helpful to me. I did have a family member who totally didn't understand ED at all. That person had the attitude that I could just snap out of it and that it was a weakness of mine. Part of me also thinks that it's damn lucky for my health team that I didn't die this last time around with ED. If the roles were reversed, I would have put myself in the hospital. I had been hospitalized several times in my twenties and early thirties, but I wasn't nearly as sick as this last time. I'm really lucky.

*

CHRISTINE BASTONE
Christine is a 49-year-old living
with binge eating disorder

I don't know that any of them even know that I have an eating disorder, so they don't connect my health with it. I've been lucky that people haven't really commented on my weight or my eating. In fact, the only one I even remember is a coworker who once commented on the unhealthiness of my eating when I was pregnant. She was concerned about the nutrition my baby was getting though, not my weight, how much I was eating, or any type of consequences for me.

*

LISA BRUNS
Lisa is a 52-year-old living
with binge eating disorder

My physician attributed my weight to my physical problems. My family never talked to me about my weight or how it affected my life.

*

LYNDA CHELDELIN FELL
Lynda is a 50-year-old living
with binge eating disorder

As an obese person, I shied from going to the doctor. Not only was I ashamed of my size, but I was humiliated each time the clinic nurse asked me to stand on the evil scale. Further, she didn't merely see my weight, she documented it. Becoming a permanent part of my record, it was like a tattoo that couldn't be erased. And the physician? Not only did she never mention my obesity or potential health threats, but she never looked me in the eye. The overall attitude was that if I didn't care enough about my health to shed weight, then why should he? I felt invisible to my physician—until I shed one hundred pounds.

As a thin woman, my physician treated me like a real person. That mentality toward obesity isn't exclusive to the doctor's office. Across all societal standards, female intelligence, good morals, and strong work ethic aren't enough. Beauty and thin body habitus continue to reign when it comes to female careers, friends, and societal worth. No wonder my eating pendulum swung wildly for so many years. One end of the spectrum held all the triumph; the other end held ugly defeat. It wasn't just me who was off balance; it was all of society.

*

JUSTINE HILDEN
Justine is a 27-year-old living
with binge eating disorder

I used to be ashamed of telling people about my eating disorder. But I have since become very open about it. When professionals who don't know me begin talking about my weight, about being obese, about losing weight, I am very open about sharing that I am in an outpatient program, and that I am getting support. At times they give me the spiel about losing weight. It's hard. I've left the facility feeling angry, sad, and upset. I know they are doing their job, but it's hard being reminded of something I've struggled with every day. Do they not think I wanted to lose weight? Do they think that I've not tried? Do they know how triggering it can be to talk about my weight? Even those who are professionals have no idea.

My friends and family have been supportive as they have gone through this process with me. They have asked questions that upset me. "Why can't you just eat healthy?" "Why can't you just diet?" "Why do you still struggle with this eating disorder so many years later?" "How long until you are in recovery?" They are questions that most people would ask, should be able to ask, and go through many people's minds, but they can be hard to hear, especially from those close to you.

I am able to answer those questions now. I am able to be okay with those questions. It's taken time, but I want others to ask questions. I want them to learn and be aware. I hope I can be the person who helps them better understand not only my eating disorder, but eating disorders in general.

*

LYDIA KENYON
Lydia is a 22-year-old living
with anorexia nervosa

Once, a few years after I had pretty much given up on ever recovering (this was approximately 2013) my mom asked me to go see a doctor, and I agreed. That doctor tried to push me into an inpatient facility and basically told me I was killing myself and needed to listen to her or else I would die. Look at me now! I didn't go to an inpatient facility (though that doctor threatened me and told me I would be committed involuntarily if needed), and I chose recovery on my own, at my own pace. Maybe not necessarily the smartest thing to do when your life is being held in the balance, but I firmly believe I had to choose recovery for myself for it to actually work. And it is working.

*

REBEKKAH KOONS
Rebekkah is a 29-year-old living with
an eating disorder not otherwise specified

Only my primary care physician talked to me about my eating disorder, and the therapist she recommended. My mother now says that the family knew but didn't know how to help. She knew I was on medicine that I seemed too young for, and would always say, "Your heart is a muscle; your body will start eating away at it."

*

MONICA MIRKES
Monica is a 58-year-old living
with binge eating disorder

I couldn't believe it when my doctor said the word "obese." That hit me like a ton of bricks. It wasn't enough for me to change my eating habits, though. My attitude was what the hell, guess I'll be fat the rest of my life. Family and friends didn't say anything to me. It was like the elephant in the living room; everyone pretended everything was fine with me.

*

RUTH PAPALAS
Ruth is a 58-year-old living
with binge eating disorder

I'm sure that behind my back many individuals have discussed it and decided that my binge eating contributes to my other health issues, present or forthcoming. No one really says much to me about it to my face. I can say something like "I really should lose some weight." Someone may respond with "Well, you know what to do." Of course I know. I can read as well as anyone else that excess weight contributes to most diseases and health issues. If you google a health issue, about the first thing it mentions is losing weight, or obesity, or what type of diet to follow to avoid or fix whatever ails you. When you visit a doctor though, he is mostly concerned with what prescription will fix or prevent the problem. Knowing that you should eat properly, and actually take the time to prepare nutritious meals, are two entirely different things.

*

DEBBIE PFIFFNER
Debbie is a 56-year-old living
with anorexia nervosa

For the most part, the doctors have correlated the health problems I currently have with my eating disorder. The doctor I see now is extremely supportive. He cheers me on when I'm doing well, and if I'm slipping he shows a lot of concern and compassion. I feel that he understands and does not blame me. I had several other health professionals who were not so supportive. I had a substitute therapist one time when my regular therapist was off. She actually said to me, "Debbie, it's time for you to grow up. You're an adult now." I was too stunned to speak, but was thinking, "Okay, so having an eating disorder is childish—something an adult would never have?" Luckily, I never had to see her again.

A medical doctor I saw for a short time told me that I didn't have enough fat reserves on my body and, if I ever got really sick, I would probably die. When I told him I understood that, he responded by telling me that from his position, it appeared that I didn't really care. I had to take a step back and tell myself that he really didn't understand eating disorders nor how I was feeling. I have seen therapists over the years who claim to specialize in eating disorders, but don't really seem to have the knowledge. One therapist whom I saw within the last couple of years after my eating disorder returned handed me a paper that was filled front and back with food items. She proceeded to tell me that this is what I should eat every day. Needless to say, that was my last visit with her.

My family did blame me. They did not provide much support or try to understand. I was thought to be looking for attention. Of course my parents were scared of losing me, but other than making sure I got the medical treatment I needed, no one ever sat down and had a conversation with me. No one in my family EVER discusses my eating disorder. If I bring it up, it's quickly dismissed. Thank God I now have a support system in my husband and my friends.

*

DENISE PURCELL
Denise is a 50-year-old living
with anorexia nervosa and bulimia

My family and I aren't close because it was such a dysfunctional family, and everyone had his or her own demons. They really weren't and aren't involved in my life to know what I've been through. Just my daughters. They know and they are supportive. And yes, I am teaching them not to repeat any of my bad behaviors.

*

HADDI TREBISOVSKY
Haddi is a 29-year-old living
with anorexia nervosa

To my recollection, there was no one who openly correlated my eating disorder with any of my health issues. To my recollection, no one really even knew I was struggling with an eating disorder.

*

Begin today. Declare out loud to the universe that you are willing to let go of struggle and eager to learn through joy.

SARAH BAN BREATHNACH

*

CHAPTER ELEVEN

Facing Food Prep

If you really want to make a friend, go to someone's house and eat with him. The people who give you their food give you their heart. -CESAR CHAVEZ

Connection to food is universal, and eating is necessary for the survival of every species. In humans, grocery shopping and food prep are closely tied to a family's lifestyle and daily routine. It's how we care for our spouse and children, and is often a symbol of our culture and faith. So how do we engage in providing for our families when we've lost touch with how to care for ourselves?

*

JUNE ALEXANDER
June is a 65-year-old living
beyond anorexia nervosa

Today, the challenge of grocery shopping and food preparation is fully pleasurable, and emotions are self-nurturing. Today, I love food, eating is a pleasure, and my body tells me what nourishment it would like for the next meal. My body and self are one. The anticipation, preparation, and eating of every meal and snack is a daily delight. I love wandering around my garden, harvesting fresh vegetables or herbs in the lead up to evening meal preparation; picking and eating fruit from the trees in my orchard; shopping and selecting groceries; going to restaurants and on picnics. I love, above all, meals shared with family and friends.

Having a healthy relationship with food helps me to have a healthy relationship with myself and with others. And vice versa: healthy relationships, food, and me; we build on and with each other. Today I enjoy full-cream milk in my coffee and on my cereal, I enjoy eating rhubarb sweetened with real sugar, I eat lollies (candy) with my grandchildren, I pour gravy on my meat and vegetables (yes, meat as well as vegetables!). I love eating ice cream as a treat, and I enjoy scanning restaurant menus for the meal that appeals to my body's needs right now. Decisions are made on feelings rather than rules. Today my relationship with food is relaxed and intimate. What I eat becomes part of me. As already stated, I listen to my body and it tells me what it wants. I love this! But for more than forty years, during my eating disorder, my mind was flooded with rules in an effort to keep the monster at bay. Shopping would require knowing the caloric value of every item put in my trolley.

Every meal was an ordeal, sandwiched between layers of anxiety and guilt. I admired anyone who could eat a meal and be happy; I marveled that they could do this. Why couldn't I? Guilt would haunt me. My meals were regimented and consumed hours of thinking time.

I despaired that I would never escape debilitating food thoughts or know when I felt hungry or full.

One of the worst feelings with an eating disorder is that something is missing, and of feeling weak to be giving in all the time. For me, failure to fill this hole within automatically translated to confirmation of incompetence and of being worthless. Finding the will to fight on when lacking confidence to make sensible decisions was challenging. By my mid-forties, after years of therapy with my psychiatrist and minister, and reflection in my diary, I no longer had deep depression. I understood the difference between genuine human experiences of disappointment, imperfection, and uncertainty versus the illness translation of those into *fat* and *unworthy*. But I was not *there* either. I had to cross the line.

My diary, 1989: *I have to complete this last leg. Of living knowing inner peace of being what I want to be, of using my energies in a positive way, of waking up and welcoming the new day and knowing I have not binged and made myself ill the day before; of being able to give to others the freedom given to me.*

STRATEGIES

Positives: My diary was slowly evolving from a survival tool to a method for building self. An early strategy was to focus on aspects of me-in-my-life that I knew were positive. For instance:

- I love people. I dislike injustice. I have a strong empathy for other people and the problems they might encounter (or the joys).
- Many people say I am bright and sunny, often smiling and helping them smile too.

- My life revolves around family, work and church, trying to do my best at each, and being nurtured by all three in return.

- I am generally organized, efficient and reliable.

- I enjoy my job. It is reassuring to know I am sane enough to work, and be financially independent.

- I am trying to like and love myself, and make a little time for myself, and do something for myself daily, something I enjoy. Likewise, I am trying to give myself the right to avoid, without feeling guilty, events that, and people who trigger feelings of uncertainty and vulnerability.

- I have to accept that the level to which I succeed depends on myself: the extent to which I am prepared to step out in faith will largely determine the extent to which I grow as a person.

Negatives: Total honesty was essential (no secrets allowed), so negatives were acknowledged, too:

- Having suffered anorexia and bulimia, I remain a sensitive person, easily exploited, and prone to feeling unworthy and inadequate.

- Food remains a challenge, and when emotional needs reach a critical point I either binge to numb my mind or starve in a bid for control.

- I have difficulty defining and putting my needs first in decision-making but am working on overcoming these pitfalls with my psychiatrist and minister, opening up and sharing with friends and family, and reading helpful books on faith and identity.

Emerging insight: I made lists for self-improvement.

- Allow time to write my memoir.
- Work on letting nothing disturb balance of self.
- Develop deeper relationship with God.
- Focus more on situations, causes and people who provide reciprocal emotional and spiritual fulfillment.
- Make time to nurture all needs—emotional, intellectual, spiritual, physical—so am best placed to help others meet their needs.

The lists became more refined and practical:

- Mix more socially, for instance in church community; seek healthy diversions to avoid urge to withdraw into shell.
- Relax with and enjoy my children.
- Do handcrafts such as cross-stitch and needlepoint.
- Allow twenty minutes of physical exercise daily such as walking, running, swimming, bike riding, with children or friends when possible.
- I love animals and adopted a kitten, Silvester.
- Read more books, especially about real people who have surmounted obstacles and can inspire me.

On reflection, these lists revealed promising intention, but putting them into action did not come naturally. The entrenched eating disorder had been the central driver of thoughts and behaviors for most of my life, so every self-love activity was laced with guilt. I could see what I needed to do to be *me*, but could not yet feel or relate to it. In many ways I had to start over in learning how to live. To heal, authentic behaviors and thought patterns for daily living had to be restored, and sometimes manually and consciously re-learned. Only then could I resume a self-driven path.

To be me, I had to stop hating food and start loving it. To be free, food could no longer be the boss that determined my moods, my everything; it had to transition from self-harm bully to nurturing and supportive self-love collaborator. I was weight-restored, but food intake was irregular and thought patterns continued to be food-driven. What else could I do? A breakthrough occurred when my therapist suggested I focus on getting in touch with my feelings, and "food will gradually take care of itself."

Regular, nutritious meals daily were essential; sounds easy, but the pattern of overeating one day and restricting the next ran deep. To overcome this entrenched behavior, I had to look beyond the food into parts of self that ED had kept disconnected for years.

The eating disorder had caused my body and self to being like strangers, uncomfortably and suspiciously sharing the same skin. The diaries provided stark evidence of this. Under the therapist's patient guidance, I began to leaf through the layers, many containing long-held secrets, to grieve (for the repressed me), retrieve and reunite with my true emotions. Basically, I began to learn to think in ways that were compassionate and authentic, and develop these healthy thought patterns to the point where they became automatic, replacing the eating disorder thoughts. This took a lot of practice.

My diary, 1990: *I see now, after much reading, that I need to give up my control with food—I must give up dieting and cessation of bingeing will follow automatically. I must not use food as a control mechanism. I MUST let it go.*

My diary, 1991: *I believe the key to curing my eating disorder is to respect myself in every way, including energy intake with food and drink. I'll look after my total health by having enough sleep, nutrition and exercise, will learn to manage my time and put myself first.*

My therapist provided another suggestion: "Separate your thoughts from those of your eating disorder." How would I know if a thought was authentic, belonged to ED, or influenced by prescription drugs? The diary would help me work through this confusion, which would remain until I quit being a slave to ED.

My diary, 2006: *I must focus on solving my problems, and refrain from using food to cope with intolerable situations.*

Read more about the diary as a self-help and therapeutic tool in my book *Using Writing as a Therapy for Eating Disorders - The Diary Healer* (http://bit.ly/24IOF5S).

*

OLIVIA ANTHONY
Olivia is a 44-year-old living
with anorexia nervosa and bulimia

I feel really fortunate because I am currently on the other side of my eating disorder. I am able to shop for groceries with the intention of eating foods that nourish me. I do love sweets, though, and realized that each day I need to allow myself something sweet so I don't feel deprived. When I was in the thick of anorexia, I enjoyed shopping and making meals. It was fun to make food for others to eat. But it became a struggle when I was so starved that I couldn't think clearly to even understand a recipe.

During bulimia I was embarrassed shopping. I bought so much junk that I was sure everyone knew I was going home to binge and purge. It was a struggle preparing meals, because I wanted the food, but knew I would purge it. I felt like I was wasting food and it was a waste of space.

*

CHRISTINE BASTONE
Christine is a 49-year-old living
with binge eating disorder

I don't actually do very much grocery shopping. My husband does that most of the time, although I make up the grocery list. That is certainly no easy task! The biggest challenge with making dinner for my family has nothing to do with my eating disorder. It's finding something that they like that is so difficult. My other challenge with food prep also has nothing to do with my eating disorder. It's having enough energy, and feeling well enough to do so. Feeling awful physically makes food prep extremely difficult.

Another challenge with grocery shopping is trying not to spend too much money. Thankfully, we have been on food stamps for a number of years. But trying to make that amount last all month while feeding a hungry family of four is difficult, to say the least. And while I do absolutely love junk food, I also like a number of things that are nutritious and good for me. But it is a sad fact of life that junk food is cheaper. Many foods that are good for me are simply out of my price range, and have been for a long time. Even with what we do buy, I have recently found out that it's probably a good thing that I don't regularly do the grocery shopping. I am about go into shock every time I see exactly what the prices are, and what the total comes to when we check out!

*

LISA BRUNS
Lisa is a 52-year-old living
with binge eating disorder

I hate grocery shopping. I know what I'm supposed to eat, but it's difficult. At times I just want to grab a burger and blow everything off. I've struggled with my weight my entire life, and basically I'm just tired. I'm so tired of this battle.

*

LYNDA CHELDELIN FELL
Lynda is a 50-year-old living
with binge eating disorder

For years I lived with the notion that if we were out of junk food, then we were out of food, even if our cupboards were full. My concept of groceries was very skewed. It didn't include fresh fruit or vegetables. My grocery list consisted of highly processed foods, including lots of sweets, ice cream, chips, sugar-laden cereal, and candy. I'm ten years into my food sobriety, and now I can see how sick that was mentally, and how damaging it was physically. But at the time it was how my brain worked. Junk food was my heroin. When the kids were little we lived from paycheck to paycheck and, as a family of six, we were sometimes strapped for cash. I wrote checks at the grocery store anyway, knowing my bank account was empty, just to get my fix. Because I ran out of ice cream.

Food prep consisted of whipping up batches of sinful treats or elegant desserts. Or making nachos or other types of comfort food. Although I took great pride in mastering a couture dessert that garnered plenty of praise from others, and my family marveled at my culinary and confectionary skills, it was all about comfort. The creamier the food, the richer the dessert, the more abundance of junk food, the more content I felt. Until I ate, and then the self-loathing and shame began.

*

LYDIA KENYON
Lydia is a 22-year-old living
with anorexia nervosa

At the grocery store, I find myself grabbing the low-fat container or with "xxx calories" plastered on the front. This was a huge hurdle to try to sail over. I can't say I did it gracefully. My dietitian was adamant that I get rid of all my diet food. I'm not sure if this is typical or not with anorexics, but I considered those foods my special foods. I had my low-calorie yogurt and no one else I knew ate them, so they were mine. I ate frozen diet meals while others ate Stouffer's lasagna. Everything I gravitated toward was lite or low-fat. It was the only way I could feel okay about eating. I think my biggest triggers are probably still having to see those products at stores and choose to buy the regular version instead of the diet version. I still slip up sometimes. It's definitely a recovery win for me if I am able to pick out the full fat version and get through the checkout with it!

*

REBEKKAH KOONS
Rebekkah is a 29-year-old living with
an eating disorder not otherwise specified

I never had groceries in my apartment when I lived alone. I felt so lost in a grocery store, like I didn't belong and everyone around me could see it. It's part of my anxiety and agoraphobia as well. On the weekends I stayed in my apartment and ordered food online. I couldn't even call, because I felt like they were judging me on my big order because I needed food for the whole weekend. There were only three places to choose from, so the delivery man knew me well! I don't cook, I don't prepare food unless you call microwaving preparing food. Mostly, I would eat unsafe food if I had some wine, because it relaxed me and I remembered how much I loved eating.

*

MONICA MIRKES
Monica is a 58-year-old living
with binge eating disorder

I stopped going to the grocery store. Simple. If I don't see it, I can't eat it. Not being busy is my trigger; if I'm not doing something I will graze. So I have picked up all kinds of craft projects! Don't know why, but if I'm just sitting around I will eat. If I'm working on a project, I stay so focused that I forget all about food.

*

RUTH PAPALAS
Ruth is a 58-year-old living
with binge eating disorder

My biggest challenge in grocery shopping is once again trying to get my money's worth. If something is on sale, even if I know I shouldn't have it, there's a good chance that I will buy it and eat it. My daughter asked me why I never make cookies or cakes. I told her that I just can't. When I make them, I eat them. When I used to bake a cake and cut a piece, I would eat it. Then I would look at the cake and the line would be crooked, so I would cut off another sliver. I can sliver a cake to death! If I baked cookies, I would first have to eat all the broken cookies. After that, none of the cookies were safe until they were all gone. I removed all the cookie sheets and cake pans from my house. I can't trust myself.

*

DEBBIE PFIFFNER
Debbie is a 56-year-old living
with anorexia nervosa

When I first developed anorexia as a teenager, I lived at home with my parents and did not have to deal with any grocery shopping or meal preparing. My mom did all the shopping and cooking, and she never wanted any of us to help. So at that time it was an issue I never really had to deal with. When my eating disorder returned in full force several years ago, I was married. Since I am no longer working and my husband has a physically demanding job, I do the grocery shopping and all the cooking. I don't really like to eat. I eat mostly to put on weight and get healthy. It can get extremely difficult for me to go into the grocery store, be surrounded by all this food, and try to make decisions on what to buy and what I might want to eat, but mostly what my husband would like to eat, since I have very little interest in eating.

For a variety of reasons, I don't go out much, and I especially don't like to drive in our Minnesota winters. We have several grocery stores in our area that let you shop online and have your groceries delivered to you. It's ideal in some ways, because I just have to pick out the exact item I want. I'm not faced with tons of overwhelming decisions. Should I buy this? Or maybe I should get that. When I do go to a brick and mortar grocery store, I tend to take a list and get in and out as fast as I can. My anxiety can become extremely overwhelming after I've been shopping and I can become angry, irritable and not pleasant to be around.

When it comes time to prepare a meal, I'm the one making the decision of what to prepare, and once again my anxiety can be devastating. I'm trying to decide what to cook for dinner, and none of the items in the freezer seem appetizing to me, so I make decisions based on what I think my husband would want. Once again I become angry, irritable and filled with anxiety. My husband always tells to me to buy and make what I want to eat. He has told me and anyone involved in my treatment that he will eat whatever I decide to buy and cook, since he believes that will help me to eat.

I wish I never had to deal with food. I wish I enjoyed eating like most people seem to. I'm not a very good cook, and I don't like to cook. I don't know what would really change that, and most times I really don't know how to handle the emotions that accompany grocery shopping and eating. It's not a pleasant experience for me. I know that my husband would do the shopping if I asked him to, but I feel I should be doing the shopping and cooking, because he works hard all day, while I am at home. I feel like it's part of my job as a homemaker. And, of course, I don't want to admit defeat. My goal is to grocery shop and prepare a meal like a normal person would. Although I may never get to that point, I will always strive for it.

*

DENISE PURCELL
Denise is a 50-year-old living
with anorexia nervosa and bulimia

Grocery shopping is hard, because while I'm buying all healthy foods, the voice in my head says, "Come on, just one doughnut won't hurt you." So I hurry up and try to get out only to revisit later and end up giving in. I will buy something and hide it, and eat it when no one is around. I used to have so much willpower; it seems that has taken a vacation.

*

HADDI TREBISOVSKY
Haddi is a 29-year-old living
with anorexia nervosa

Calorie counting was never a struggle for me, and because I was in high school and college during my ED years, grocery shopping and food prep didn't really factor in as a trigger. There have been times as an adult when grocery shopping or food prep felt overwhelming even outside of an ED, and there has been a temptation to buy all junk food or just skip a meal out of the mere frustration that comes with deciding on what would taste good or what would be healthy. I'm not sure if this is a remnant of my ED or just my personality, but I find that sometimes eating is a chore for me. Yes, there are foods I thoroughly enjoy and will eat happily, and that happens more often than not, but there are days and times when absolutely nothing appeals and I have to force myself to eat so I don't get sick (migraines and headaches, typically). This makes grocery shopping and food prep difficult.

CHAPTER TWELVE

Braving Restaurants

The food that enters the mind must be watched as
closely as the food that enters the body.
-PAT BUCHANAN

Restaurant dining is an indulgence that promises relaxation and
pampering. But for those struggling with an eating disorder, it
presents unseen challenges. Portion sizes, the number of choices, and
even the environment can easily lead to anxiety and feeling
overwhelmed that then become a trigger. What are your challenges
when invited to dine with family and friends?

*

JUNE ALEXANDER
June is a 65-year-old living
beyond anorexia nervosa

During my long-term eating disorder, it was easier to eat at home.
At home I could eat what I considered safe foods, and regulate the
amounts. The problem with eating out was that it was full of

unknowns, and unknowns made me feel very anxious and afraid. Later I would be plagued with guilt and would feel more isolated and misunderstood, due to people around me not understanding that my behaviors were due to an illness and not due to the real *me*. When dining out was unavoidable, I would tend to starve myself all day, and exercise excessively, to appease ahead of time the guilt that would come with giving an impression of being normal and polite, and with consuming unknown food items that might be presented, and which I could not avoid without appearing rude.

This excerpt from my memoir, *A Girl Called Tim*, illustrates the difficulties faced as an eleven-year-old with anorexia.

Each May and September school holidays, for as long as I could remember, I set traps to catch rabbits, which were a pest. In the past year, Dad had shown me how to set snares for kangaroos and wombats as well. My latest rabbit catch became a stew. Mum knew I loved the tender, fresh meat, more so because I'd hunted and gathered it myself, but now I refused to eat it.

She was angry. "Why won't you eat, who do you think you are?" Then, with Dad in the washhouse, scrubbing his hands and combing his wavy hair as he always did before coming to the table, she said, "If you don't eat, I'll tell your father, and you know he has enough worries already." Mum was always telling me about Dad's worries. We had too much rain, not enough rain; too much wind, not enough wind; butterfat prices were falling, superphosphate prices were rising; in autumn the cows' milk was drying off too early, in spring the cows were blowing up with milk fever; all year round, machinery was breaking down. I felt the burden of my parents' worries, but couldn't eat the rabbit. The guilt would cause me to run for miles along the rocky river track, and eat only a crust of bread and half a tomato the next day.

At the end of September, I began my final term at primary school and was exercising three hours a day. With my thinness more apparent, my mother tried to persuade me to swallow a vitamin mixture. I refused. I hated the smell and feared the calories.

Sometimes she became very upset. One afternoon after school she insisted I accompany her to visit an old friend Mrs. Banks, a widow, several miles around the corner of our valley. Anyone who lived just outside our valley was referred to as being "around the corner." I didn't want to go, my thoughts were screaming at me not to go, but Mum promised, "We'll take a bunch of flowers and stay only a few minutes." In the car, on our way there, she revealed that we were invited for afternoon tea. Dismayed, I said, "But I need to be home to do my jobs." "Don't be impatient, and don't be rude," she warned as she pulled up beside Mrs. Banks' wooden picket fence. Mrs. Banks was waiting at her front gate to greet us. The flowers were presented and admired, and we wandered as slow as snails around Mrs. Banks' pretty garden on our way into her cottage. I tried to suppress the urge to run. Then came the dreaded "Come inside and have a cup of tea." In we went, and I sat on a chair beside Mum at the small kitchen table, struggling to keep still while the two women chatted. Wood was fetched, and the fire stoked to help the kettle boil. It took forever. I politely declined the offer of a glass of milk or a glass of sugared cordial. Mum glared. I said, "I'd like a glass of water, please." Things deteriorated fast. Mrs. Banks offered a plate of homemade biscuits and cake. I wanted to escape. I could feel my cheeks going beetroot red as I said, "No, thank you, Mrs. Banks." Seething at my poor manners, Mum accepted a biscuit with her cup of tea. The chat continued.

"Mum's angry, but I can't stay here," I thought. She was about to get angrier because suddenly my hands, on which I'd been sitting, broke loose and I began squirming on my chair, swinging my legs and folding and unfolding my arms. I nudged Mum while Mrs. Banks refilled the kettle. "I want to go home," my eyes begged. "Sit still," she flashed back.

Mrs. Banks returned and conversation continued. Suddenly my anorexic thoughts took over. I stood and blurted, "I want to go home to help Dad in the dairy." "Just a few more minutes," Mum smiled sweetly. Veiling her annoyance, she said the biscuits were so crisp and crunchy, she would eat another one. Pleased with the praise, Mrs. Banks offered to write out the recipe. Mum and her neighbors were always swapping recipes. "Thank you, Alice. I'm sure Lindsay will like them," Mum said. "You stay for your recipe and I'll walk home," I chipped in, thinking this was a good time to make a break and the walk would compensate for the time I was seated. But Mum stood too, smiled and said to Mrs. Banks, "I'll get the recipe another time. We'd better go home now."

The truth was, Mum couldn't bear the thought of me walking home along the road. She'd worry a neighbor might drive by and see me running. I was an embarrassment. I raced out of the house to the car. I stood beside the passenger door and hopped from one foot to the other while Mum and Mrs. Banks dawdled, with Mum choosing a few plant cuttings to strike for her garden. The farewell at the front gate took an eternity. At last Mum opened the car door and sat behind the wheel of our black FJ Holden. She was angry. "How dare you?" she raved as she drove us home. "You can't sit still for half an hour. What's got into you?" She didn't know I had anorexia. She didn't wait for an answer before continuing, "You were good. Now you are rude. Everyone will be talking about you and your bad manners. You always want your own way. Why don't you think of others?" On and on she went. I said nothing. She would not believe I did not want to be difficult, that my mind was being overtaken by thoughts that were not really me. I wanted to get home and run, run, run to make up for all that horrid sitting down.

One Sunday a few weeks later, I was invited to play with a school friend, Louise, at one of the grandest farmhouses around. The invitation included Sunday lunch. I didn't want to go and said I preferred to wander in the bushland and look for wombats sunning themselves on their mounds, or watch lyrebirds doing their dance. "You have to go," Mum said, distraught. She didn't know what was worse: declining the invitation or making me go and risking further embarrassment. "You must go," she said, exasperated. Joy upset her, and now I was upsetting her too. It was impolite to turn down invitations.

"I'll run away if you don't go," she threatened. Sometimes when my sister was rude, Mum ran out the back gate, slipped through the house paddock's wire fence and disappeared up the gully. She always returned after a few hours, but I silently resented my sister for being horrid. My sister back-answered, shouted, swore and poked her tongue at Mum. I didn't understand why, preferring to avoid the house so I didn't have to listen to the noise. I tried to be good so as not to cause sadness. But now Mum was threatening to run away because I didn't want to go out for lunch. Somehow finding the courage to override the urge to stay at home, I said, "Yes, I'll play with Louise and stay for lunch."

I rode my bike the one and a half miles to Louise's house, the last four hundred meters being a dusty dirt track bordered by a cypress hedge. We had time for a play before lunch so we climbed the hedge, trying to get all the way through, from branch to branch, without putting our feet on the ground. By the time the lunch gong sounded we looked and smelled like little cypress trees ourselves, with sticky green bits in our hair, inside our blouses and over our woolen jumpers. Exercise was good, but my day was about to deteriorate badly.

The Morrison family, one of the region's earliest settlers, had a big dairy farm and employed a share-farmer to milk their cows. Louise and her two older sisters and parents lived in a big cream-brick house surrounded by a rambling cottage garden.

Every child in the district loved going to birthday parties at Louise's house. We played games like "Pin the Tail on the Donkey" and "Drop the Hankie" before sitting down to a brightly decorated table laden with party food. There would be jelly set in orange quarters, macaroons so light they almost floated away, hundreds and thousands sprinkled on *quarters of buttered bread, dainty squares of hedgehog, marshmallow in ice cream cones, and hot sausage rolls. All were homemade.*

Until now I'd felt special, being invited to birthday parties and Sunday dinners as well. That was before anorexia developed in my mind. Now I was filled with dread. Sunday dinner loomed like a heavy black cloud and there was nowhere to hide.

Louise's mother was a great cook but a stout and scary, no-nonsense woman. Louise had confided several times how she'd had her mouth washed out with pepper for telling fibs. Now I sat at the kitchen table with the family, a plate loaded with slices of roast beef, baked potatoes and pumpkin and boiled peas, drenched with rich gravy, before me. I felt I was before the firing line. Fearful as I was of Mrs. Morrison, I could eat only the peas; terrified, I ate them slowly, one at a time, trying to avoid the gravy. There was no opportunity to shift food into my pocket. So I shifted it around on my plate, and pretended to eat, but I was fooling nobody. Looking downward, sensing everyone was staring at me, my face turned bright red. I wanted to disappear under the table. "This is the worst meal in my life," I thought. "Everyone has finished eating and is waiting for me." At last Louise's mother removed my plate. "What a wasteful child," I knew she was thinking.

Without a word, she served dessert. Big bowls of jelly, custard and preserved peaches, topped with a blob of thick cream fresh from the dairy, were passed around the table. Normally I would love this but now studied my bowl with a sinking heart. The jelly and custard had been sweetened. The peaches were submerged in syrup. Louise's dad and her big sister cleaned their bowls and left the table. Her mother was clearing the table and washing the dishes. I sat, too scared to move, apart from my swinging legs, out of sight under the tablecloth. Louise sat beside me. At last we were shooed outside. Relieved, I didn't want to stay a moment longer and said, "Got to help Dad with the cows and calves."

I feared that Louise's mother would phone Mum and tattle. Sure enough, as soon as I entered our backdoor Mum lectured me on my pig-headedness and poor manners. Blow Louise's mother, I thought. She had phoned to ask my mother if I was sick, but I'm sure she inferred I was just plain rude. I couldn't wait to go outside to start my jobs and to be alone with the bossy thoughts in my head. Mum did not make me go for meals at anyone's house again.

At age twenty, newly wed (excerpt from A Girl Called Tim):

One Saturday George's mother invited us to lunch with family visiting from interstate. We gathered on the Coster (his family's) homestead's front lawn, in the sun, against a backdrop of shady camellia and peppercorn trees. A red and white gingham cloth spread over a trestle table, set up on the veranda, was barely visible beneath platters of ham, chicken, creamy potato and Waldorf salads and buttered bread rolls. I rapidly calculated that I could eat several lettuce leaves, two tomato slices and half a boiled egg. I was struggling for control, and strict calorie counting was vital to avert anxiety. Everybody was piling food on their plates and I marveled at how they could eat and not think twice about it. The aunts and uncles were kind, but in asking about my accident they said, "You are looking well." I had binged the previous night and their comments confirmed I was fat. I began withdrawing from conversation to deal with my thoughts within. Pavlova, pineapple cheesecake and trifle, each piled lavishly with freshly whipped cream, were served for dessert. Everyone was eating at least one serving.

George's mum loved preparing and eating rich food. Her desserts were delicious, and the guilt of declining to eat any added to my self-loathing. I felt increasingly suffocated, trapped. "I do not belong. I do not want to be here," my mind was screaming. "I need to escape." I whispered to George, "I want to go home. Now." I felt removed from, and uncomfortable with, the warmth and love around me. Things came to a head when George reluctantly left the family gathering to return me to our house. He yelled and I howled. "You could have waited until we had a chance to have a chat with our visitors," George said. "They will think you are rude and self-centered." "I can't help it," I shouted, hating myself, and bursting into tears. George had no hope of being able to understand, because I was unable to explain. He disappeared back to his family.

*

OLIVIA ANTHONY
Olivia is a 44-year-old living
with anorexia nervosa and bulimia

Eating with family or friends wasn't much of a challenge. I didn't have family nearby, except for my son. It wasn't until he was older when he would make comments about my eating the same thing again. If I was in a bulimic phase, I just made sure that I ate a small portion of whatever the meal was. I then purged if I felt I had too many calories that day. I was such an isolator with my marriage to ED that I really didn't have to eat with family or friends much.

*

CHRISTINE BASTONE
Christine is a 49-year-old living
with binge eating disorder

My biggest challenge around dining with family or friends is probably waiting to eat whatever meal it is, or then waiting to go home so I can binge. An additional challenge is the energy that it takes. At home, if we do not have guests, I can lie down and eat in my room. Yes, I know eating while lying down is not good for my digestion. But I don't care, because it certainly helps to conserve my limited energy.

*

LISA BRUNS
Lisa is a 52-year-old living
with binge eating disorder

I eat little to nothing. I don't like anyone seeing me eat. I feel like I'm being judged. I'm the sister who had weight-loss surgery, and that still couldn't help me lose and maintain a healthy weight.

*

LYNDA CHELDELIN FELL
Lynda is a 50-year-old living
with binge eating disorder

Eating out was a treasured time. I certainly wanted to get my money's worth, and it afforded the perfect excuse to indulge. Further, I wasn't alone in my indulgence at the table, so I felt no shame. We learn quickly which restaurants serve large portions, way more than our stomachs should handle in one sitting, yet the voice in my head wanted to be sure I got my money's worth. Couture restaurants serving tiny portions at large prices were avoided, because what was the point? For me, it was all about the quantity.

Going to a restaurant now has a totally different angle for me. I'm there to enjoy time with family and family. I stick to healthier menu options such as roast chicken, and eat very little of the accompanying side dishes bursting with carbs. I might indulge in a margarita, but I always skip dessert.

In the early stages of food sobriety, I had to be very strict to avoid falling down the rabbit hole. Now, ten years in, I can relax a little bit in the restaurant setting. My dear sweet hubby and I are now empty nesters, and I travel frequently for work. Today I can indulge while traveling without threat of entering my danger zone. When we return home, I go right back into my healthy eating habits. It's when I fall off the wagon at home that I find myself in quicksand.

*

LYDIA KENYON
Lydia is a 22-year-old living
with anorexia nervosa

Right now I don't have quite as much aversion to new foods and restaurants that I used to. It's still there, but for the most part I am confident I can find something adequate on the menu to satisfy me. Sometimes I even surprise myself by trying something new. The only thing that might make me feel better and more comfortable about eating at home is knowing that my food is prepared in a way that I approve. I'm trying to move past that, but it's still a struggle. At least now I am able to go out and have fun without panicking half the day trying to make sure we go to a restaurant that I know has "safe" foods.

*

REBEKKAH KOONS
Rebekkah is a 29-year-old living with
an eating disorder not otherwise specified

I remember being offered lasagna at my sister's bridal shower. I said I had already eaten, and held the plate and pretended to eat. But suddenly I had to go and quickly put the plate on the table and hoped no one noticed. At rehearsal dinner, I managed to eat the big dinner but later excused myself so I could purge. I was happy my family saw me eat, but the food wouldn't be sitting in my stomach all night.

*

MONICA MIRKES
Monica is a 58-year-old living
with binge eating disorder

If I do eat at a restaurant, I'll make two meals out of it. Half there, the other half for lunch the next day. Definitely easier at home, and less temptation for me. I have no willpower.

*

RUTH PAPALAS
Ruth is a 58-year-old living
with binge eating disorder

My challenge is that I want to try everything and eat ALL of what tastes especially good. Sometimes when I find myself overeating, I feel that those I am eating with are judging me and my food choices and consumption. It doesn't stop me from eating, it just makes me feel bad. I've always belonged to the "clean plate" family. "If you don't clean your plate, you don't get dessert." I loved dessert. Even at restaurants, when the server asks, "Would you like to hear about our desserts?" I have to respond, "I didn't clean my plate—no dessert." Or maybe even worse, I overate and dessert won't even fit down my throat!!

*

DEBBIE PFIFFNER
Debbie is a 56-year-old living
with anorexia nervosa

As a teenage with an eating disorder, I hated eating at home or out with anyone around. I knew my eating habits were different, and I also knew that people, especially my family, were watching me closely. I ate alone when possible, but as a teenager I was required to eat with the family, and it was extremely difficult and anxiety-provoking.

Now I'm very comfortable eating with people around, both at home and at a restaurant. When I first started my recovery this time around, my husband watched me carefully whenever I ate. If I was having a snack, he'd always ask what I was eating. The natural reaction to that was to stop eating so I could maintain that control, but I knew in my heart that it was just out of concern for me, and that he was trying to support and encourage me. But it's that control issue, and I had to fight hard against it.

At this time in my recovery, I would much rather eat out than at home. That way, all I have to do is pick something off a menu and try my best to eat it all. There is very little thought put into it and not an overwhelming number of choices to make. Now I would actually rather eat with someone than eat alone. I do, however, tend to put enough food on my plate when others are around so that people will see that I can and do eat a proper amount of food.

*

DENISE PURCELL
Denise is a 50-year-old living
with anorexia nervosa and bulimia

When the holidays are around and people offer me cookies, I tell myself I don't want them and am not going to eat any. But that doesn't work. While in front of people, I'm good and will decline, or have little at dinner. At home, the urge comes up and I'm bingeing again.

*

HADDI TREBISOVSKY
Haddi is a 29-year-old living
with anorexia nervosa

When I was in the middle of my ED, my emotions and challenges involving eating with family and friends varied, depending on who I was eating with. Initially, my ED was born out of the teasing I endured from my middle school boy peers, and so when I ate with them at lunch I decided that to avoid teasing I could simply skip that meal. When I had boyfriends, I never ate in front of them, insisting I wasn't hungry. This was a challenge, because often while on a date I was actually hungry and would end up with a headache, spoiling the date in the end. I was very self-conscious about what I was eating, especially in front of pretty peers or boys I was interested in. In front of my family my challenges were different, because I was mostly just trying to hide the fact that I had an ED while also trying to limit what I was eating in front of them.

*

Your present circumstances
don't determine where you can go.
They merely determine where you start.

NIDO QUBEIN

*

CHAPTER THIRTEEN

Navigating the Holidays

> People are always judging you based on where you're from, where you went to school, how you look, how you talk. But at the end of the day, you're going to have to look into the mirror and accept who you are. It's all about being authentic. -ANDRE CARSON

Holidays are a stressful time for many, but especially so for those struggling with an eating disorder. Many holidays are centered around food and eating, faith and culture, and often present triggers for both ends of the eating disorder spectrum. What holidays are hardest for you, and how do you cope?

*

JUNE ALEXANDER
June is a 65-year-old living
beyond anorexia nervosa

Christmas was always the most difficult time for me, due to unresolved family secrets and issues as much as coping with food on the plate. Pretending everything was fine and sunny was expected;

anything deeper than this was not tolerated. My attempts to seek answers would be sharply dismissed ("That happened a long time ago," "You are the only one who thinks there is a problem, get over it"). For years my depression and anxiety, and therefore my eating disorder thoughts and behaviors, would intensify in the lead up to the festive season—like, this time of the year was a reminder of wounds within that yearned for understanding and healing within the family circle.

For decades, Christmas lead up was a time of dread, because to heal from my eating disorder, secrets that stemmed from my early childhood had to be painstakingly located and revealed. Regaining an authentic life required embracing the truth. Without family of origin support, this task was harder to achieve, but achievable nonetheless. Countless times I backed out; the task was too scary, it was easier to live a chaotic, uncertain and tormented part-life. The eating disorder's thoughts mocked me; they screamed that sharing my dreadful secret, "You have to be stupid if you can't eat three meals in one day," would lead to incarceration, being locked away, losing my children. In this way, eating disorder thoughts encouraged and demanded silence. They reduced life to a shallow and fragile pretense. Outward efforts to appear super-organized and capable, thinly veiled the inner fear and torment. Eating disorder thoughts hissed that sharing the inner struggle would land me in a mental hospital, where I would be alone, and confirm I am nothing. So I had to push beyond this, and eventually, by reaching out to, and trusting, people who believed in me, beyond the illness, I gradually reintegrated my true self, and became free to enjoy holidays and being free.

Following are the strategies used to regain myself and embrace ongoing healing:

- Without fail, eating three nutritionally-balanced meals and snacks daily. Food is medicine.

- No calorie counting, and no weighing.

- Employment can provide a sense of purpose and self-worth at a time when nothing else does.

- Being candid with understanding family members, as they provide ongoing support.

- Keeping a journal and listing positive things done during the day, like planting seedlings, baking a cake, phoning a friend.

- When anxious, dividing the day into quarters. Making it to 10:30 a.m., and writing down how I am coping, again at 1 p.m., and so on.

- Repeating affirmations, such as "Action beats anxiety" and "I deserve to be treated with respect," at times of stress.

- Accepting that prescription drugs, while causing side effects, are at times essential.

- Separating myself from my illness. This self-awareness strategy helped me to recognize and avoid people and situations that enabled my illness.

- Imagery is helpful. I pictured a raw egg, with the yolk my soul and the white the world around me. No matter what goes on in the white, protect your yolk. Don't let it scramble.

- Being my own best friend. Would I want to bruise my best friend? No!

- Asking: Does this thought belong with my illness, or with me? If with illness, hit the delete button.
- When feeling vulnerable and confused, reaching out for and accepting guidance from trusted others.
- Attending to feelings diminishes food as an issue.
- Embracing the moment with friends and family of choice; having fun!
- Walking by the sea with my dog, or cuddling my cat. Embracing and connecting with nature in its many forms is food for the soul.
- Facing a stressful situation or fear often brings a reward in an unexpected and delightful way.
- Acknowledging a right to be born and to live is empowering.

The diary is potentially a great teacher. The challenge is to learn its lessons. Sometimes I write multiple entries in one day. This is usually when an anxiety-provoking situation is about to occur or has occurred. I prepare for what seems a challenging event, like a soldier going into battle, as self-preservation is my priority. Through the process of diary writing, strategies are considered and put in place; later, after the event, the diary enables a debriefing.

*

OLIVIA ANTHONY
Olivia is a 44-year-old living
with anorexia nervosa and bulimia

I would say that Christmas brought the most anxiety regarding food. There was just such a long stretch of time with all kinds of temptations. I am happy that I'm not currently restricting or purging. My strategies are allowing myself treats. Daily treats! I also try to eat nourishing meals. During my last healing, I really studied up on things. I love saying that butter is a health food! I spent so many years thinking fats were the enemy. They're not!

*

CHRISTINE BASTONE
Christine is a 49-year-old living
with binge eating disorder

My challenges in relation to the holidays are not much different than dining out. The only added dimension is that I miss my youngest sister, Liz (who died by suicide in 2012), more on the holidays or at least notice her absence more than I do on days that are not holidays.

*

LISA BRUNS
Lisa is a 52-year-old living
with binge eating disorder

The holidays are horrible. I refuse to cook, because I know I can't or shouldn't eat the unhealthy food. My sister continues to make her holiday favorites and bring them to my house. I guess the whole family shouldn't have to suffer because I can't control my eating. Last Thanksgiving my niece made a pie. I ate some despite the family telling me not to eat because it was going to make me sick. I ate it and immediately got sick, and stayed that way after everyone had left.

*

LYNDA CHELDELIN FELL
Lynda is a 50-year-old living
with binge eating disorder

The holidays were similar to the restaurant setting, in that there were absolutely no boundaries or limits. The festive cookies, decadent desserts and holiday candy were adored, and the voice in my head reasoned that each holiday comes only once a year, so I better enjoy them while they're here. Holidays were an excuse to come out of hiding. A two-pound chocolate Easter bunny would disappear within a day. Valentine's meant heart-shaped chocolates tormenting me with various fillings. A one-pound bag of holiday M&Ms could disappear within an hour. Fourth of July and three-day weekends meant potato salad, potato chips, barbecued meats slathered with savory sauces, corn on the cob dripping with butter, and other comfort food. It wasn't that these foods were eaten only on these dates; it just meant that I could eat them without hiding. So holidays were a time when I could enjoy decadent food without the shame. That is the definition of freedom for someone living with binge eating disorder!

Ten years into my food sobriety, the holidays remain hard. I adore the scent of cinnamon, cloves, warm sugar cookies, and pecan pie. Our family expects traditional meals using traditional childhood recipes, including my dad's favorite cookies, my mom's sausage dressing, and creamed sweet potatoes adorned with toasted marshmallows, along with an assortment of other comfort food. Last Thanksgiving our youngest son came home from college and made a batch of my favorite mint bark. I allowed myself to have a nibble, and ended up eating five pounds. I became physically ill and emotionally ashamed. I regained control, thankfully. When our son came home for Christmas break a few weeks later, he made another batch. I didn't allow myself to have nary a crumb. Not. One. Single. Crumb. It was just too risky.

*

LYDIA KENYON
Lydia is a 22-year-old living
with anorexia nervosa

Thanksgiving. I don't really like any of the traditional foods, except for bread rolls, so it's difficult, because ED is already telling me not to eat and I have to fight that and myself. I think I got through the last several holidays very well. In regard to food, my feelings were a mixture of fear and excitement. I talked them through, and blogged about them during the experience. This was the first year in about ten that I was able to feel somewhat "normal" for Thanksgiving and Christmas, and it felt so good.

*

REBEKKAH KOONS
Rebekkah is a 29-year-old living with
an eating disorder not otherwise specified

Holidays were not so tricky for me, as I come from a huge family and we were always bustling around, catching up with one another and holding the newest babies. One time, we all sat down and my mom blatantly said, "I hope you're not getting an eating disorder." My fake laugh was some of my best acting. Little did she know that I had been living with it for years at that point. I don't blame her, but if she had rephrased that to "Honey, are you okay? You're not eating," I might have opened up more. But that's not how my family functioned, and at the time I was grateful, because it meant I never had to get better.

*

MONICA MIRKES
Monica is a 58-year-old living
with binge eating disorder

Since meeting my goal weight, if I do eat the wrong foods, I have to take the next few days to really monitor my food choices. It is a give-and-take system for me, and I understand this.

*

RUTH PAPALAS
Ruth is a 58-year-old living
with binge eating disorder

My biggest challenge at the holidays is that there are so many favorite things to eat. I don't want one of each cookie—I want a whole dozen in one sitting. I don't want one helping of turkey, homemade stuffing with gravy, and homemade cranberry sauce— I want to eat until no more will fit. It seems that on holidays, people prepare things just for me. "We knew this was one of your favorites, so we made it special for you." I feel guilty if I don't eat that item, and guilty if I overeat that item to show my appreciation.

*

DEBBIE PFIFFNER
Debbie is a 56-year-old living
with anorexia nervosa

When I was younger, all holidays provoked anxiety. I knew everyone would be keeping their eyes on me to see what I ate and how much. And on holidays like Thanksgiving or Christmas, there was just way too much food, and the anxiety of having to choose what and how much I was going to eat could become absolutely overwhelming. I did not look forward to any holidays, and with my family even the smallest of holidays was centered around food.

At this point in my recovery, the holidays and the food served don't provoke anxiety, unless I'm the one who is hosting, which, fortunately, happens very seldom, since we have a small house with a small kitchen and no formal dining area. If I do host, it's usually just meat, cheese, buns—premade items I can pick up and serve buffet style. Very little thought has to be put into it, therefore minimizing the grocery shopping and cooking anxieties. If I'm invited to someone's home for a holiday meal, I just take what I want, and I no longer worry about whether anyone is watching. It is a more pleasant experience than it was the first time around.

*

DENISE PURCELL
Denise is a 50-year-old living
with anorexia nervosa and bulimia

Christmas is the biggest holiday. It's not at home so much but visiting family with their goodies and more goodies, so pretty soon the day is a wash anyway, so why shouldn't I have some more? Then the guilt and disgust begin, so I have to purge or else sink into depression even lower and not want to venture anywhere. If I could sleep, that would be my coping. I don't cope. I just sit in a seat of hate and disgust, and feel that I should hide under a rock because I'm so detestable.

*

HADDI TREBISOVSKY
Haddi is a 29-year-old living
with anorexia nervosa

As far as I can recall, I had no particular challenges or emotions in relation to the holidays. I know that this is a very common time for folks to stress over what they eat, ED or not, but I truly can't remember a time when the holidays invoked anxiety regarding food for me.

*

CHAPTER FOURTEEN

Finding Good Treatment

My worst days in recovery are better than the best
days in relapse. - KATE LE PAGE

Although eating disorders are physically and emotionally destructive, each journey is highly individualized, making treatment challenging. Whether one seeks individual or family psychotherapy, medical care and monitoring, nutrition or medication, in certain cultures and social circles, a stigma remains about seeking treatment at all. What treatment have you sought and responded to, if any?

*

JUNE ALEXANDER
June is a 65-year-old living
beyond anorexia nervosa

At age thirty-three, in early 1984, after a night of self-harming, I phoned for an urgent appointment at the local health clinic; my regular doctor was away, but a new doctor was on duty. Desperate, I saw him, and that appointment made all the difference. This new doctor saw my problem was more than physical symptoms, and wrote a referral to a city psychiatrist. Getting the referral, as my diary noted, was indeed a promising event, but the subsequent seven-month wait for the appointment became another trial, for by now I was in a suicidal frame of mind.

My diary, June 1984: *I cannot go on like this. Too much stress, strain. If I eventually get to see the psychiatrist, well it will be very good if he can help me...otherwise I might as well die. That's how I feel. I'm crying out for help, but who can help? It's been so long since I was able to eat like a normal person.*

Other health professionals had tried their best but to no avail, to the point where the new doctor had surmised, "Professor B is the one man who can help you." Regular appointments would be required, and this meant relocating from the country to the city several hundred miles away. This was a big undertaking, with no promise of recovery, and with employment to find, housing to organize, and four children to settle in a new school.

By the time I met the psychiatrist, whom I called Prof, in late 1984, I was thirty-three, caught in a steep downward spiral of self-destruction. I had developed anorexia nervosa at age eleven, and this illness was embedded in my brain. Prof won my trust, and saved my life. For years the thought of my next appointment with him provided a lifeline of hope. He became my recovery guide, mentor and confidante.

Prior to my first session with Prof, I worried he would conclude there was nothing wrong with me, thus confirming that I was an incredibly inadequate person. I had been seeing other doctors for five years. Despite their efforts, through misdiagnosis my struggles had gotten worse. Perhaps I was a hopeless case. However, within minutes of meeting Prof, I knew he could help me. He saw beyond my illness, and confirmed that I had an illness in my brain and perhaps, just perhaps, with the right help, I could overcome it. I definitely, immediately felt relieved. Surely his words meant that I was not simply a weak-willed person after all. "You have never been helped since developing anorexia," Prof said, giving me a long life history questionnaire to fill in, and asking me to keep a diary of everything I ate and my moods each day. He suggested that my private diaries, kept since developing the illness at age eleven, might help to sort my problems.

My second appointment, in four weeks, seemed a long way off. At this next session, Prof provided the first real diagnosis of the illness that had been plaguing me since childhood. He confirmed I had developed anorexia nervosa and now bulimia nervosa, and described my condition as "fair." He said, "Your life has been full of anxiety and depression." I was a chronic case. Prof wrote out a prescription, the first of many over the next several decades.

There was no quick fix. I was in the preliminary bout of fighting my illness. There was a long, hard haul in front. The enormity of this struggle hit me as I left Prof's consulting room that day and I wondered, not for the first time, if problems in my mind were too entrenched. However, on my next visit Prof said, "You're not to give up hope. You've had the illness more than twenty years and it will take time to get well." I became determined to show myself, and Prof, that I could be fathomed, that I could cure myself with his help.

Acknowledging that thoughts and behaviors, which for a long time have seemed helpful, if not absolutely essential, must be let go because they are harmful, not authentic, and symptomatic of a brain-based disorder, is beyond scary. I faced the challenge of accepting that my structure of self, to which I had devoted and sacrificed many hours of each day since childhood, was false and deceptive. Creating a safe and sound structure for self was made more difficult when support from my family of origin was not forthcoming. I felt rejected and misunderstood when I tried to confide, and they suggested that I was wasting my time. "Why are you still seeing that doctor? If he hasn't cured you yet, he can't be any good." Another time, "How can you say you have an illness when you are able to work full time?" My family did not understand that a mental illness is not a choice and has no fixed healing period. They did not understand that it is possible to be high-functioning and productive in others areas of the brain, just like someone who has a broken leg can continue to use his other limbs and be productive and purposeful. Misunderstandings like this only served to strengthen the eating disorder's voice.

Prof was the prime member of a small team in whom I developed trust and faith. He understood, and set about helping me dig through and confront, the layers of illness that were suppressing the true me. Reluctantly, I gradually stopped telling my family of origin that I was seeing a psychiatrist. Perhaps my illness had been entrenched too long for them, for they did not respond to my invitations to share in my healing journey. I had to change, to live, but they saw no need to be part of this process. After all, they said, "You are the only one with a problem." I yearned for deep and meaningful discussion, but conversations became limited to the weather and other inconsequential topics. As years passed and I became more "me," I became alienated from the family circle. Locating the threads of my identity, and separating them from the thoughts and feelings that belonged to my eating disorder, without family participation and support was painstakingly difficult.

Visits to Prof took on a pattern. I would arrive with pages of handwritten or typed notes, which I would pass to him, and nestle in the big comfortable chair opposite him while he read my ramble. Then he would look at me, ask questions, make suggestions, offer guidance, check prescriptions. He believed in pharmacological solutions but also understood the value of narrative medicine. The medications slowed my illness thoughts, allowing time for the gradual restoration of self-belief chiefly through the mode of written communication. Prof understood that I felt safer writing what I didn't yet feel able to voice. In this way, the diary provided a tool with which we built a trusting relationship, a vital first step in reconnecting with self.

In addition to overcoming the fear that accompanied eating three nutritious meals and three snacks daily, the locating and re-integrating fragments of self into a sound foundation, from which to venture forth and re-engage in life, was a mammoth task. It included the tedious process of dealing with and letting go of thoughts, behaviors and relationships that fed my illness.

I remained in unhealthy and chaotic situations and relationships, which Prof called "mistakes," for years, too scared to let go. The eating disorder bully had been part of my life for so long that being kind to myself, and keeping myself safe, made me feel uneasy. As soon as I started to feel safe, I would be drawn into fresh chaos, for that was familiar. Prof, kindly describing many of my choices aligning with the eating disorder traits as not right for me, patiently offered renewed encouragement: "It is not that you are wrong but that solution (or person) is not right for you; keep trying."

My authentic self slowly became aware I was making decisions that were maintaining my illness and keeping me a prisoner. The problem was that my attachment to making decisions which maintained chaos and turbulence, was as strong as the entrenched attachment of my illness to me. In my quest for freedom, I had to develop sufficient skills, self-awareness and self-belief to recognize, confront, resist and defuse the inner chaos of illness thoughts and behaviors. Only then would I be able to resist the pull of outer chaos and settle into an environment that was safe, secure and stable.

Over time, my diary helped me to recognize and accept that I needed to ask for help when the niggling, disruptive thoughts began— the earlier the better, for a slip as simple as eating a small chocolate bar to suppress a feeling of rejection, could snowball into a relapse that might last for months. The diary helped to clarify true thoughts. Besides providing a method of communication with Prof, and remaining a place in which to confide, it also became a medium for reaching out.

Drawing on my diaries in letter writing to Prof helped me to edge forward in recovery, by providing an avenue for connecting with a person of trust, even when I didn't know which way was forward, and from this tenuous leap of faith, to slowly begin to trust and connect with the true me.

With Prof's encouragement, I also began to read through earlier diaries, and reflect on them. This involved revisiting painful and traumatic times, but now I had a trusted person with whom to release and share them, and to re-story memories too difficult to process. I cried for the lost young June. I wanted to take the eleven-year-old's hand and shepherd her along a safe and well-lit path. Instead, I had to keep turning the pages, watching years slip by while she became more and more entangled and lost in the dark forest of the eating disorder. Digging through and addressing layers of suppressed emotion was a prerequisite to releasing her from the eating disorder's grip and to constructing a safe base of self-belief. I found it helpful to create notes of specific thoughts and feelings, between appointments, and reflect on and organize them further, to discuss during my next appointment with Prof.

Gradually, over several decades, the combination of therapy, medication, and love of my children, their dad, and friends instilled me with sufficient courage and trust to let the eating disorder go, and with it the shame and stigma that had clouded my thoughts for decades. At the end of the day, Prof could do only so much: the extent of healing was up to me. I had to reach the point where I could transfer my belief and trust in him to belief and trust in myself, to be free.

Besides Prof, my support team grew to include a general practitioner, dietitian, neurosurgeon and minister of religion. Every now and then I told Prof that I believed I was *there* now, and insisted that he supervise cessation of the latest pharmacological medication. Prof would comply, but skeptically, and say, "I am not giving you a green light; your light is showing amber; my door will remain open for you."

For several months I would try living without his guidance and without the medication for my eating disorder and comorbidity anxiety and depression, but my authentic self remained fragile. Unable to eat three meals a day without being overcome by debilitating fear, guilt, and anxiety, I would soon fall into a black pit, lacking sufficient skills and self-belief to make decisions that were in my best interest. Other members of my treatment team would encourage me to resume taking the medication and assure me that to do so would not be a sign of weakness, but rather an expression of self-love and caring behavior toward the young girl June. Prof would welcome me back, his gentle guidance would resume, and my healing journey would continue from where we had left off.

The year 2006 was the first year in more than four decades that was not dominated by my eating disorder. By now I was eating three meals and three snacks daily, and no longer slipped into deep depression or felt overly anxious. Able to function and engage more in mainstream life, my thoughts turned to a long-held desire of writing my memoir. Turning this dream into reality would require the reliving of those lost decades I would rather forget. However, I felt ready for the challenge. Mental health problems would continue, but my foundation of authentic self was sufficiently strong now to withstand this ultimate test.

As a first step, under Prof's guidance over a seven-month period, I eased off all medication. I had been taking antidepressants and other prescribed drugs for more than twenty-five years, the latest without a break for nine years, and I wanted to be free of all of them, to be totally *me*, while writing my book.

Prof encouraged me to write my story, but warned that even a small reduction of medication by xxx milligrams one month at a time could cause my health to regress. So we proceeded slowly, slowly; I practiced self-care, wrote the book, and a cathartic release of emotion, accompanied by a surge of deepened self under-standing, ensued.

Prof was a great teacher and encourager. My memoir, *A Girl Called Tim*, was released in 2011. By this time our relationship was transitioning from that of psychiatrist and patient to one where our roles merged, leading to enriching academic and mental health advocacy discussion. I became less a patient and more an author, writing books to help raise awareness of eating disorders and disseminate findings in the eating disorder research field for health practitioners and people affected by the illness. I looked forward to these discussions with Prof. He sometimes exhibited cynicism about the release of new findings and treatments, and his insights inspired me to think as an observer rather than a participant in the mental health system, and to look and inquire beyond the obvious. For instance, he suggested that some new treatments that I mentioned were like a new chocolate bar, just presented in a new wrapper with a new name. "That treatment has been around for years," he would say. What mattered most was not the treatment so much but the level of trust formed between therapist and patient.

Over the years, Prof patiently taught me many useful techniques to strengthen authentic thoughts. If feeling caught in a bind a problem, today I automatically think action beats anxiety and, in making a decision, ask myself what is in my best interest? If feeling unworthy, or experiencing self-doubt, I remind myself to stand tall and own my space, for I deserve to be treated with respect.

Perhaps the most important lesson Prof taught is that life is not fair. I felt incensed at the injustice of this statement when he bluntly pronounced it during one of our many sessions. But when I pushed aside the eating disorder's interpretation, and absorbed the meaning of his words, I found them to be helpful and liberating. I had been expecting life to be fair; indeed, often doggedly insisting that it "should be." It wasn't, and there was no universal dictate that it need be.

Expecting perfection, and everything and everyone to be right and just, had fueled anxiety and set the scene for continual disappointments. My eating disorder loved it. Getting hung up on an issue, usually in relation to family, employment, or mental health care, because it wasn't fair, had served only to strengthen the eating disorder's hold, as it found yet another "reason" for me to binge or restrict, or engage in other self-harming behaviors. I began to see that the black and white, inflexible and isolating rules of the eating disorder were not sustainable, and I learned to love the many shades of gray.

Prof taught me to love and treat myself as I would a best friend. In my darkest moments, when I feared I would lose the love and respect of my four children, and even the right to have them live with me, Prof encouraged me to tell each of them, at every opportunity, that I love them. These were words I had longed to hear, but did not hear from my own parents. So I tell the June within, who has grown into an adult now, that I love her too. My children are in their forties now, and I continue to tell them I love them at every opportunity. Prof knew that unconditional love has a healing power all of its own.

Read more about the importance of trust in the therapeutic relationship in *Using Writing as a Therapy for Eating Disorders - The Diary Healer* (http://bit.ly/24IOF5S).

*

OLIVIA ANTHONY
Olivia is a 44-year-old living
with anorexia nervosa and bulimia

I've had many different counselors over the years. I've also been in inpatient treatment. The least helpful form of treatment was going inpatient in the psych ward. They didn't have an actual eating disorder program. It was basically what you would expect any random psych ward to have. Men and women were there who were suffering from various mental illnesses. My primary care physician visited me in the mornings to see how I was doing, but I had zero therapy or help. It was basically just a place to give me lots of meds and meals. And I didn't eat them. I refused to eat. So they put me in a room with all glass walls to watch me. It was not helpful at all. I had a seizure, thankfully my only one. I ended up leaving the hospital without any tools or help given. I didn't fully regret a separate time in the psych ward, because I admitted myself for getting help with a self-injury problem (I still had ED, but was really struggling with cutting). They prescribed a medication that took all the good feelings that I got from cutting away from me. But as for getting help for ED, the psych ward failed miserably. I also went inpatient to a hospital that had an ED program. That was helpful to an extent. They had counselors there to talk with. They also had different art activities to do. It was also helpful because I met one woman whom I became friends with who is also a mom.

I left earlier than advised, because my son was little and I felt guilty for being away. And I had a new determined attitude to heal from ED. I didn't want to be like some of the women in that hospital. It seemed like some of them didn't truly want to heal. I wanted a life. I wanted out from the grip of ED. I was determined to get healthy with a new therapist and dietitian. For me, inpatient was best for helping to break the cycle. Once that cycle was broken, I did better working with my team at home. It was hard to focus while in the hospital, because I missed my son so much. If I had been an inpatient while in high school or college, it might have been more beneficial for me.

For me, seeing my therapist once and sometimes twice a week, plus going to my dietitian twice a week really helped. I also regularly saw my physician. They were my team and I trusted them. They really were so helpful. I loved them! I did feel like I failed them years later when I relapsed. I lived in a different city. So I got the name of a counselor from my doctor. Thankfully, I loved my doc and counselor.

I was so lucky again! What really helped me get well was journaling throughout my journey. I did that each time I struggled. But this last time I did it through my private blog. My counselor read my posts the day of my appointment so that she would have a fuller picture of how my life had been since my last appointment. That really helped! Then I didn't have to catch her up, and in addition, typing out my feelings as I was going through them was much more enlightening for her than my verbal words could ever express in fifty minutes. For me, seeing a therapist whom I really clicked with, plus a doc who listened and truly cared were most helpful in this last round with ED. I think I should have been in the hospital, though, to help break the horrible cycle I was in. I think I was truly lucky that I didn't die.

*

CHRISTINE BASTONE
Christine is a 49-year-old living
with binge eating disorder

I haven't had any therapy or been to any treatment centers regarding my eating disorder. I have had some experience with them regarding my depression, though. I personally haven't found therapy to be very helpful. I find a lot more help from books like this one written by people who have been there.

I have also had some experience in psychiatric wards of hospitals. I have found those to be more helpful than therapy. Although, surprisingly, I found the other patients to be at least as helpful as the staff. Not that the staff wasn't helpful. Then there's the enforced routine of eating at mealtimes and sleeping at night, plus a kind of protection from the outside world. Those things are helpful too. The medication may or may not be helpful. But I think it's best to find this out while in the hospital rather than right after being discharged!

The first time I was discharged from a psychiatric ward, the medication kicked in with unpleasant side effects shortly after. As this made me sleep thirty out of thirty-six hours, my hard-won routine was very effectively destroyed so soon after I had to go back to reality. The second time, I insisted on staying in the hospital until the medication kicked in. That time I found the side effects to be pleasant. My appetite was reduced, and I had all this energy! That time I was able to keep to my hard-won routine for a while. The right medication and the part-time outpatient hospitalization program I attended for a few months really helped me make the transition between the hospital and my reality, otherwise known as "the real world."

*

LISA BRUNS
Lisa is a 52-year-old living
with binge eating disorder

I was going to therapy and it seemed to work, but I am unable to go now because of family obligations. I have issues that I can't control, eating being one of them.

*

LYNDA CHELDELIN FELL
Lynda is a 50-year-old living
with binge eating disorder

Because obesity is often seen as lazy and lack of self-control in many cultures, for a long time the only treatment prescribed was admonishment along with caloric restriction and exercise. In the 1990s, appetite suppressants became popular but did little to reduce the growing obesity epidemic, because they did nothing to address the underlying mental issues. Nonetheless, pharmaceutical companies raked in billions from diet pills until a combination known as fen-phen later proved to have adverse cardiac affects. Bariatric surgery then became popular because it reduced the stomach size. A second surgical option reduced the absorption of nutrients by bypassing part of the small intestine. Medical advances now offer four surgical options for obesity. Like many, I was naturally curious about this new "miracle" option for losing weight. But intuitively I knew that surgery ignored the underlying issue. It was merely a bandage—not a cure.

Over the years I tried every diet under the sun. I even attended Weight Watchers with some success. But it never lasted, because I always felt denied. Diet was a four-letter word, and meant starvation, deprivation, and torture. It meant I couldn't have what I needed most: comfort. As one of four sisters, and with a weight-conscious mother, diet was involved in many conversations. The very word evoked feelings of dread. Many different diets were tried, and all promised magical results but were actually out of balance. I remember one diet when we were allowed only pineapple and mangoes for the first two weeks. We were told that the diet would clean out our gut and pave the way for weight loss and better health. Although I didn't like mangoes and the diet sounded a bit crazy, I followed it to the T, and lasted two weeks. I hate mangoes to this day.

When gastric banding became available, I considered it many times. I simply felt I needed a magical fix, and then I could handle it from there. Although there was something horrifying about the whole idea behind it, I also envied those who were courageous enough to go for it.

In the end, success was found in my own regimen. When I weighed xxx at the doctor's office that fateful day ten years ago, it was like a switch flipped in my brain. But I refused to call my new regimen a diet because it had only one rule: whatever I put in my mouth had to be nourishing. I didn't count calories, I didn't weigh portions, I didn't worry about balancing proteins and carbo-hydrates. I just ate for health. It was a true lifestyle change. I also began walking with my neighbor two to three miles from Monday through Friday. Each month I lost an average of xxx pounds.

I don't judge those who find success using whatever means are available to them, but my personal journey was to seek better health overall. Shedding the obesity has impacted my health in many wonderful ways, which is why I work hard to maintain it. I've fallen off the wagon a few times, and when I do it's a tremendous struggle to find my footing. The usual self-loathing and shame soon follow a single sinful indulgent. Now I use that as my moral compass: a few moments of chocolate melting in my mouth simply isn't worth the days of shame.

Now that binge eating disorder is considered a mental issue, I'm hopeful that those of us living with it will soon have better options from which to find freedom from the illness.

*

LYDIA KENYON
Lydia is a 22-year-old living
with anorexia nervosa

My first experience wasn't great. My mom made some calls, and I was very young and confused. I had no idea what path to take or what would benefit me the most. I went to a hospital about an hour away, and began outpatient treatment, but got a little put off when the dietitian put me on a very intense diet that put me in the hospital with what I now know was refeeding syndrome. Fast forward several years, and I grudgingly agreed I needed help, so my mom contacted a woman she knew at the doctor's office here in town, and got me an appointment. I went on some antidepressants and just kept maintaining. I saw several doctors and therapists during this time, but nothing really stuck. Finally the bills were getting high, and my parents said I had to start pitching in. So, I quit seeing anyone, and pushed recovery even farther onto the back burner. I was on and off for years. I always had this gut-wrenching guilt, knowing that what I was doing wasn't healthy or productive, but I was trapped. I couldn't stop my behaviors on my own, but I didn't know how to ask for help.

Finally, in September 2015, I knew that the only way I could get better was to ask for assistance. After months and years of fighting it off, I made a few phone calls and got in touch with a woman who was there with me about halfway through my journey, until the bills got too high. She told me she was more than happy to begin seeing me again, and I went from there. I now have a wonderful team including a medical doctor, therapist, and dietitian who each play their part in helping to keep me on the track to recovery. And the best part is that they aren't experts. They are new to this too, but willing to learn beside me, because I am ready to do the work. One huge thing that has been so helpful in my recovery is not focusing on body mass index, or calories, or weight. Numbers are my enemy, so I let the professionals take care of that.

*

REBEKKAH KOONS
Rebekkah is a 29-year-old living with
an eating disorder not otherwise specified

I was referred to a therapist by my primary care provider when I opened up to her about restricting my eating. At first I was excited to go. I hoped she would be a listening ear, but I didn't want her to truly help me, I just wanted someone to listen. So when she tried to teach me tools, I stopped going. Looking back now, I know that the whole point of therapy is to try to learn tools to cope and to not restrict, but at that time I wasn't ready, and I just wanted someone to listen.

*

MONICA MIRKES
Monica is a 58-year-old living
with binge eating disorder

After spending money for several programs that did not work, I had resigned myself to just being unhappy with my weight. While attending a Christmas party I saw two friends, a mother and daughter who had both lost over a hundred pounds each! What miracle had been performed? They had found a treatment center with a doctor who understood and recognized how important it is to see results

214

quickly. I thought, sign me up! This man explained, really explained, how the body works and what we were going to do to together to make positive changes.

*

RUTH PAPALAS
Ruth is a 58-year-old living
with binge eating disorder

I haven't sought therapy or any treatment centers. I have self-diagnosed and have seen some doctors. I hate to have it on my medical record that I have a problem, because it could be seen as a pre-existing condition, and who knows what that could lead to?

*

DEBBIE PFIFFNER
Debbie is a 56-year-old living
with anorexia nervosa

I have been in and out of therapy for my eating disorder. I think therapy can be extremely helpful, if the therapist is truly qualified and has experience. And most important, that they are willing to listen, because everyone who has an eating disorder has similar issues, but everyone is different.

The quickest way to put me on the defensive is to not hear what I'm saying, or ignore what I'm saying in favor of what they think I should be thinking or feeling. What I found least helpful with therapy is the reason we are here, telling our stories. We have all been through it. Although our eating disorders may be different, we are all in this together. We all have food issues, and it has affected our lives. I have seen therapists who claim to know all about eating disorders and how to help you, but in reality I have found myself on more than one occasion feeling as though I know more about eating disorders than they do.

I have heard this saying so many times, and I truly believe it: Unless you have been through it yourself, you cannot possibly fully understand it. One therapist handed me a two-page list of foods on my first day, along with the statement "I would like you to eat this every day." Are you kidding? Do you not know that if I could eat that much food just on your say-so, I wouldn't be here looking for help? I had a therapist tell me that I needed to start adding small amounts of fat, such as a tiny pat of butter to my vegetables. When I told her that I eat *anything* I want—that I put butter on everything already, she looked at me like I was out of my mind. There are anorexics who avoid certain foods or who count carbs or any number of things. I always counted calories; it didn't matter what type of food, as long as I ate only a certain amount of calories. She seemed baffled by that information.

It has been my experience that there are some therapists out there, including the one in the treatment center I attended last year, that really do not understand the full aspects of a patient having an eating disorder. On the other side, I have had therapists who were very knowledgeable and have helped in many ways. Finding the right therapist is a trial and error process.

*

DENISE PURCELL
Denise is a 50-year-old living
with anorexia nervosa and bulimia

I went to a therapist who specialized in eating disorders and we pinpointed the reasons why I felt the way I did, and why I did the things I did. But the therapy part was very hard. I had to get my parents involved, and they weren't very supportive. It was a response of "Therapists always blame the parents." Well, if the parents fit..... So I tried to continue working on just my part, but never felt validation from my parents for anything they did.

*

HADDI TREBISOVSKY
Haddi is a 29-year-old living
with anorexia nervosa

I have never been officially treated for my ED. However, I have seen two different counselors at two different times in my life, once in college and once as a married mother of a baby. I primarily sought the guidance of a professional for helping me deal with anxiety and depression. It was helpful to have a third party to talk to who wasn't directly involved in my life. I felt it was beneficial to speak openly about my struggles without worrying how that person would take it. I also found it beneficial to have a professional who knew what questions to ask me so that I could fully process the difficulties I was having coping with my feelings. The hardest thing about therapy/counseling is that in order to get better, it's up to me to put in the work. I have taken prescription medication in the past to help deal with anxiety and depression, but I'm at a point in my recovery where I prefer to cope without it, so it is up to me to maintain a healthy balance in my life (physically, emotionally, mentally, socially, spiritually) so that I can manage the anxiety and depression, and also my eating disorder tendencies.

*

CHAPTER FIFTEEN

Social Support

> Surround yourself with people who provide you with
> support and love and remember to give back as
> much as you can in return. -KAREN KAIN

Parents, family and close friends can play a significant role in supporting those faced with an eating disorder. Often their compassion and care can become a lifeline when we fail to help ourselves. What gestures or statements from family or friends have you found most supportive?

*

JUNE ALEXANDER
June is a 65-year-old living
beyond anorexia nervosa

During my thirties and forties, I developed a rapport and trust with my psychiatrist, a minister of religion, and a therapist trained in mindfulness. Gradually I gained courage to seek their guidance when feeling torn between giving in to the pull of entrenched eating disorder thoughts and daring to trust fledgling authenticity. The pages of my journal became the pebbles that formed my road to freedom. Through trusting others, I began to embrace a stable and secure me.

My diary writing today contrasts sharply with the ED-orchestrated thoughts and feelings expressed during the years lost in my illness. Today, the process of writing, particularly in putting pen to paper, helps me to sort thoughts and place them in context. The benefits of written expression have multiplied through learning techniques that help me help myself. These include mindfulness skills that assist in letting go or disengaging with negative thoughts, and cognitive behavior therapy skills that help to identify unhelpful thoughts and behaviors, and learn or re-engage with healthier skills and habits. Words tumble onto the page, without fear of interruption, misinterpretation or judgment. From there, if need be, emotions are channeled into a manageable form of communication that can be reflected on alone or discussed with trusted others. The release of troubles and doubts, or of pros and cons on anything considered important, makes way for clarity and calmness.

Fortunately, my eating disorder treatment team, recognizing that writing was a tool with which they could reach me, helped the diary progress from a means of not only survival, but also a way of healing. Furthermore, they encouraged writing as an alternative to talking or thinking. Guidance in mindfulness skills helped me to use the diary to reinforce messages from therapy sessions, and this process supported reconstruction of self.

My diary, 1990: *I see now, after much reading, that I need to give up my control with food—I must give up dieting and cessation of bingeing will follow, automatically. I must not use food as a control mechanism. I MUST let it go.*

My diary, 1991: *I believe the key to curing my eating disorder is to respect myself in every way, including energy intake with food and drink. I'll look after my total health by having enough sleep, nutrition and exercise, will learn to manage my time and put myself first.*

My diary, 2002: *(My new therapists) have helped me understand that I was born as an extra-sensitive person, and don't have a "filter" like normal people do, to protect my core, my soul. They are also helping me to see that I can separate my monstrous eating disorder from myself by recognizing which thoughts are mine and which belong to my monster, who only wants to hurt me.*

To be *me*, I had to stop hating food and start loving it. To be free, food could no longer be the boss that determined my moods, my everything; it had to transition from self-harm bully to nurturing and supportive self-love collaborator. I was weight-restored, but food intake was irregular and thought patterns continued to be food-driven. What else could I do?

How would I know if a thought was authentic, or was influenced by ED or prescription drugs? The diary would help me work through this confusion, which would remain until I quit being a slave to ED.

My diary, 2006: *I must focus on solving my problems, and refrain from using food to cope with intolerable situations.*

I was almost sixty when, tentatively, driven by an urge to learn more about the illness that had profoundly affected my life and those of my loved ones, I began to attend eating disorder conferences and began to feel understood, and to understand my illness more in the context of my life. I had an illness that made me feel worthless, that was all. Knowledge, in all forms, is helpful.

An unexpected, heartwarming outcome relating to family accompanied the sharing of my story publicly in the introduction to *My Kid is Back* (2009) and in my memoir, *A Girl Called Tim* (2011). By then, fifty years had passed since I had developed anorexia. While daring to hope for an inkling of understanding from my family of origin, this never came, but support and acknowledgment did come from childhood neighbors and family friends who wrote to say "Now we understand." The support came from outside the family circle rather than from within.

My children also were able to put their experience more in context, and to see the eating disorder in the context of what it was: an illness. As a family our unity strengthened. I owe my life to a network of support that includes my children's dad, my children and grandchildren, friends, psychiatrist, therapists, neurosurgeon, doctors, minister of religion and faith in God. While I lost my family of origin, and my marriage, I have gained another family during my healing process . . . a family comprising people from all walks of life in the eating disorder field.

This family of choice nurtures my fledgling self-belief, helps me know that no matter what happens, I'm okay. Acknowledging and respecting the person before, and beyond, the illness makes a world of difference. Acknowledgment and respect inspire hope.

*

OLIVIA ANTHONY
Olivia is a 44-year-old living
with anorexia nervosa and bulimia

For me, it was so helpful and important for my healing process to have genuine support. I honestly didn't want my family to be in my business. So, for me, this last time I was married to ED, I didn't tell any of them. My friend came over and noticed right away that I lost weight, over thirty pounds in six weeks. It didn't help me, but made me feel embarrassed and ashamed to see the look of pity on her face. She didn't mean anything negative by it, but I was really embarrassed. I kept a calorie count for my therapist, but ended up stopping that because it kind of made me compete with myself to keep the calories in that low range. For me, it was best if no one brought up ED. If I wanted to talk about it, then that was my choice.

I had my team to talk to about ED, and they were safe and trusted. They understood. It just wasn't helpful to hear people's uneducated advice, or even their concerns. I was already in treatment. I already knew I had a problem. I already knew I was playing with fire.

*

CHRISTINE BASTONE
Christine is a 49-year-old living
with binge eating disorder

Since people don't really comment on my weight, this is a difficult question to answer. But in any struggle or problem, anything that conveys understanding, empathy, support, encouragement, validation and/or love is helpful for me.

*

LISA BRUNS
Lisa is a 52-year-old living
with binge eating disorder

I didn't have anyone help me. I'm alone with my struggles.

*

LYNDA CHELDELIN FELL
Lynda is a 50-year-old living
with binge eating disorder

Because of the shame and stigma associated with obesity, and the obviousness of our condition, binge eaters rarely admit our struggles, not even to those we trust. The notion that obesity is pure gluttonous behavior coupled with lazy and slobbery remain steadfast. We buy larger clothing to hide our growing girth. We become housebound from the shame. We find ways to hide the evidence of our indiscretions when we fall off the wagon. I never received support from family or friends because I never opened the dialogue, which is critical in order for support to take place. Obesity doesn't just manifest one morning like a case of chicken pox. We don't just wake up fat one day. Binge eating is a mental illness saturated in secrecy. Further, we're caught in the crosshairs of a clinical debate: do we suffer from a form of addiction, or do we have a true mental disorder?

If I had to offer a statement about how to best support someone who suffers from binge eating, I would advise family and friends to be sensitive to our weaknesses, especially during holidays and celebrations. It's okay to have the table filled with traditional favorites, but include healthy options such as a veggie tray, greek yogurt-based dips, fresh fruit and cheese, hummus, lettuce wraps, chicken kabobs, etc. Next to the eggnog, offer sparkling water or fresh juice. These kinds of choices encourage us to eat healthy, and help us avoid the rabbit hole.

*

LYDIA KENYON
Lydia is a 22-year-old living
with anorexia nervosa

One of the things that have been so beneficial is my husband offering to make meals and serve my plate up for me. I know I would take smaller portions, and he always gives me just the right amount to push the envelope. I find myself shutting down and becoming quiet when I am worried or struggling with behaviors, so it's good for me to be around people who know me well and can see when that side of the disorder is flaring up. It's also really nice and encouraging when someone tells me how proud he or she is, especially if that person has been there with me from the beginning. I know they means it, and I'm now in a place where I can accept it.

*

REBEKKAH KOONS
Rebekkah is a 29-year-old living with an
eating disorder not otherwise specified

When I know I have gained weight or am having an off day and someone says I look good, it really helps. I used to associate looking good with being thin, but when I'm heavy I realize I get just as many encouraging compliments, and that helps put my eating disorder in greater perspective.

*

MONICA MIRKES
Monica is a 58-year-old living
with binge eating disorder

It helps if whoever you live with will be okay with not having any "bad" foods in the house. In the beginning, I had no willpower. As the weight fell off quickly, I was empowered. I could see the difference; I was motivated now! I could do it. Hell, I did do it!

*

RUTH PAPALAS
Ruth is a 58-year-old living
with binge eating disorder

Most people just don't get it, so they don't say or do anything helpful or encouraging. Since I'm self-conscious about my weight, I appreciate their saying nothing. If there's someone struggling with the same issue(s) I am, we can bond over it, and talk, and even joke about it. Sometimes we can even eat our way through it. My sister, however, gets it. We were recently in Jamaica and she wanted to take a photo of me. I said, "Please don't take a full-length picture. Nobody wants to see ALL of this!" She took a full-length picture anyway and showed it to me. She said, "I see nothing wrong with this picture! You are fifty-eight years old, smiling in Jamaica! Be proud of yourself! It is what it is." I realized she was right. This picture is found with my bio in the back of this book.

*

DEBBIE PFIFFNER
Debbie is a 56-year-old living
with anorexia nervosa

The most helpful thing people can do is support me. They don't have to actually understand what I'm going through, but they can still offer support and compassion. Accountability is very important. Right now I have a great doctor. He seems to understand what I am going through and how difficult it can be. He praises me and even jokes around with me when I'm doing well. He makes suggestions, not demands, and being accountable and not disappointing him gives me an added push to keep going. If there is a slip or I remain lateral, he doesn't chastise me or try to alarm me. He just gives me a gentle reminder to get back on track.

My husband has been supportive and frequently compliments me. I put on a pair of yoga pants not long ago and asked him if my butt looked big. He responded that it did. I then asked him if it looked huge. He replied that no, it did not look huge, just big. The other night he grabbed me by my upper arms to kiss me and said, "Wow, feel those muscles!" I said, "Nice try, but that's not muscle. It's fat." In the past, these kinds of statements may have sent me into a downward spiral. But today, because of the support and seeing the smile on his face, it's a compliment to me. My best friend recently told me how great I looked. There was a time when I would have interpreted that to mean I was fat. But because she has been so supportive, it was a wonderful compliment. I want and need to be accountable to these people. Their encouragement is more help than any therapy I've received.

*

DENISE PURCELL
Denise is a 50-year-old living
with anorexia nervosa and bulimia

I think that to understand the struggle, you need to know that it's not for attention. It's lack of understanding, self-judgment, self-harm, feelings of having no power over your life, and trying to grasp at anything you can have control over. It's punishing yourself when people say "You've gained weight," or "That model is perfect." What are we teaching? You came into this world as a perfect baby, right? No one said you were fat or ugly. But somewhere along the line life stepped in and told you what you should be, look like, act like, and you would be loved and happy forever. But that's the fairytale ending, and we all have many of those in our minds. Instead, it's a lifelong battle with ups and downs and so much stress just to think of what to make for dinner. People laugh, but I have to plan out the night before so I wouldn't mess up my weight, otherwise my mind would be free and I will eat whatever I want in multitude and then throw it up.

*

HADDI TREBISOVSKY
Haddi is a 29-year-old living
with anorexia nervosa

As I've mentioned before, no one really knew I was struggling with an eating disorder while it was happening. However, the signs that I was dealing with anxiety and depression were a little more clear. There was a time when I was at a longtime low, which lasted several months. I was on vacation with my family and while standing on the beach, a place where I should have been content and happy but clearly wasn't, my mom approached me and said she thought it might be time to try to get help or medication for my depression. I feel there can be a stigma surrounding medication use in Christian circles for mental illness, and I was definitely nervous that my parents and others I respected would look down on me for seeking help outside the church. When my mom suggested I get help in the form of medication or counseling, I felt a huge burden being lifted from my shoulders. This was an absolute turning point in helping me find some semblance of normal thinking, which helped me to finally get to a place where I felt I could manage my anxiety, depression, and ED without medication. Before that, I had been living in such dark thoughts for as long as I could remember that I didn't even know what it felt like to not want to hurt myself. I think mental illnesses can be related to one another, and in my case I believe that getting treatment for anxiety and depression helped in my recovery from my anorexia as well.

There was another time when anxiety and depression were taking the lead in my life and my weight dropped quite a bit. During this time I was already recovering from my anorexia, but as the anxiety and depression increased I was forgetting to eat or felt too sad to eat (as opposed to intentionally managing my weight by skipping meals). My dad was the one who took charge in this situation, and called for a weekly lunch date, calling it "Fat Tuesday." Of course this could be taken the wrong way for those of us struggling with an eating disorder, but in my case I knew it was just a playful way for my dad to address his concern for my clearly diminishing figure. Fat Tuesdays were when my dad would meet me for lunch anywhere I wanted (while I was in college) and would buy me whatever I wanted as long as I ate it. This is a time I will always look back on fondly, because I knew my dad was concerned for me, and so he took action instead of putting all the action steps on me. Dealing with mental illness can be crippling when you feel you don't deserve to get better. To have people in my life who will gently take charge when I can't has been life-giving.

*

CHAPTER SIXTEEN

Braving Social Advice

When we consistently suppress and distrust our intuitive knowingness, looking instead for authority, validation, and approval from others, we give our personal power away. -SHAKTI GAWAIN

In an effort to help, sometimes a well-meaning individual will offer a statement or gesture that has the opposite of the intended effect. Others might lack understanding or have a preconceived judgment about your eating disorder. What gestures or statements were least helpful or supportive during your struggles?

*

JUNE ALEXANDER
June is a 65-year-old living
beyond anorexia nervosa

Revealing your secret life with an eating disorder to anyone, even yourself, is a tough challenge for it requires exposing your inner being with no buffer for protection. Fear can cause procrastination of disclosure, because the response is unknown and might deeply affect what happens next. Sometimes when the story is shared, nobody reciprocates, or unhelpful responses rebound, ranging from "Nobody but you has a problem in this family, so get over it," to "You need to go to church more often," or "You're not the only one who is tired, you know (your father is, but he never complains)." My family, probably driven by frustration, made such comments so often that their words became etched, like tears, in the walls of my soul. Though said with the best intentions, the words stung nevertheless, bolstering the eating disorder voice and precipitating multiple regressions.

Ideally, families will learn as much as they can about the illness that has developed in their child or other family member, and learn skills to help confront the illness on their loved one's behalf. Otherwise they run the risk of supporting the illness rather than the patient, thereby making things worse instead of better, and prolonging the duration of the illness. Today, families can find support for themselves and their sick loved one through sharing their concerns in online eating disorder support groups such as F.E.A.S.T. (www.feast-ed.org).

Often it is the well-armed, informed parent who helps the family doctor see that a child's symptoms are indeed those of an eating disorder. Or in the case of a young or mature adult, the sharing of diary extracts can voice for the patient what the illness will not allow them to express verbally. In this way, a doctor may gather sufficient insight to become aware that the patient is indeed ill. Blood tests, and other clinical tests like weight checks are not alone sufficient. An eating disorder resides in the mind.

When I became involved in the eating disorder advocacy and research field, to my amazement I began to feel like I had the makings of a new family, one in which I felt I belonged. It did not matter that this was a global family, with face-to-face meetings few and far between. Acceptance, respect and non-judgmental attitudes helped me to venture more into the open and into mainstream life. Book research led to meeting experts in the field and learning about Maudsley Family Based Treatment for young people with anorexia. As soon as I heard about this, I thought, oh, I wish that treatment had been around when I had been a kid; it might have saved my family (www.maudsleyparents.org).

Looking back, I wish someone had been able to say to me before I married, "Look, that torment you feel is due to eating disorder thoughts and behaviors. This is why you're feeling this way; this is why you're acting this way. You have an illness and we can help you fight it. We can give you and your family skills. Those thoughts belong to the illness, and these thoughts are the real you; we're going to help you strengthen the real you." That would have been incredibly helpful, too. If my husband-to-be had been included in the treatment process, we are both sure our marriage would have been saved.

Read more about the importance of family involvement in my book *Using Writing as a Therapy for Eating Disorders - The Diary Healer* (http://bit.ly/24IOF5S).

*

OLIVIA ANTHONY
Olivia is a 44-year-old living
with anorexia nervosa and bulimia

In college I had a doctor who should not have been working with eating disorder patients. She didn't understand it, and was very judgmental. She was impatient, frustrated, and asked me when I was going to stop "that adolescent behavior." I felt like such a loser already. She didn't understand that it was a mental illness. She made me feel worse about myself, and as a result I restricted more or binged and purged more. The therapist I was seeing at the time was helpful to a point, but I could feel that she didn't truly understand my eating disorder either. She told me she felt like she was following me, stomping out the fires I was setting. It was frustrating. I moved out of state and didn't miss them! So for me, having judgments about what I'm doing to myself is really not helpful. It wouldn't be for anyone!

*

CHRISTINE BASTONE
Christine is a 49-year-old living
with binge eating disorder

I don't have a specific answer, but anything that conveys judgment, condemnation, dismissal, harsh criticism or ridicule is extremely unhelpful.

*

LISA BRUNS
Lisa is a 52-year-old living
with binge eating disorder

My family didn't know or didn't want to support me. I feel very much alone and have no one to talk to.

*

LYNDA CHELDELIN FELL
Lynda is a 50-year-old living
with binge eating disorder

Comments such as "You need to lose weight," or "All that weight you're carrying isn't good for you," are not only unhelpful, they are hurtful, because it insults our intelligence and appearance in the same sentence. For whatever reason, obesity seems to be associated with low intelligence, which only adds to our humiliation and shame. I have an eating disorder that affects my brain. But it doesn't affect my intelligence. Yes, I know I need to lose weight. Yes, I know all that excess weight isn't good for me. Do you think I intended to harm myself by eating that junk food? No child ever says he or she wants to grow up to be fat.

The food industry deserves partial responsibility in that highly processed foods, which generally lack nourishment, are cheaper than fresh, organic food. Those without means to drive to the grocery store for fresh food are forced to shop at the convenience store on the corner. Nothing good comes from that.

Our youngest son was born a good eater right from the start. He was always larger than his older sister. Even his feet were big.

Eventually he became obese. He was also highly sensitive to caustic remarks, as am I. When family members made comments such as "He would be so handsome if only he lost weight" within earshot of our son, the pain and shame were written all over his face. And mine. I was horrified that they would say such a thing to a child! These types of statements are designed to intentionally inflict emotional pain. Some people believe such statements can shame us out of our eating disorder. Eventually our son shed the weight on his own around age fifteen, and is now a thin college student earning a Ph.D. in physics. Was he large? Yes. Was he stupid? No. People need to be mindful of the emotional harm such statements can inflict on kids and adults. Kindness and gentle encouragement always trump over words that wound.

*

LYDIA KENYON
Lydia is a 22-year-old living
with anorexia nervosa

I know it's natural to become frustrated or upset when someone with an eating disorder doesn't eat, but that only makes me feel worse. Something that would help in this situation is talking through why I don't want to eat such and such an item, and how they might be able to help me get through the mind blocks that are happening.

*

REBEKKAH KOONS
Rebekkah is a 29-year-old living with
an eating disorder not otherwise specified

When I'm at my thinnest and I'm starting to fall back into bad habits, people saying "You need to eat," or "Why are you so thin?" are actually unsupportive. It makes me uncomfortable and I immediately shut down.

*

MONICA MIRKES
Monica is a 58-year-old living
with binge eating disorder

I really just tuned them out. There was one who was so negative with what I was doing, that she couldn't say anything positive. It is so true: if you can't say anything nice, don't say anything at all.

*

RUTH PAPALAS
Ruth is a 58-year-old living
with binge eating disorder

My first husband once told me, after I had a baby and had lost some of my baby weight, that I was fat, ugly and worthless. That was over thirty years ago, and I still hear my ex-husband and feel the feelings that went along with his statement. He did apologize and we get along now. I can forgive, but not forget.

Before I went to Jamaica, my sister-in-law told me that I could go there and feel okay. After all, you should see how people look on the beach and it doesn't matter how big they are. It wasn't so much what she said as how she said it. That was over fifteen years ago. I still think of that every time I put on a bathing suit. When a girl at church poked me in the belly and told me I needed to "lose that," I began my preoccupation about my weight. I guess I was a bit chubby but until she said something, I was unaware of it. It's possible that I may have lost weight naturally. Instead I became obsessed with my body and my weight. I think about it all the time.

I've heard hurtful comments and seen disapproving looks regarding my weight, but no one is as hard on me as me. I am self-critical. I feel like I can never have the perfect body. Some people said that if I lost weight, I would be healthier and happier (like I didn't know that). Unfortunately, neither they nor I knew I had an eating disorder.

*

DEBBIE PFIFFNER
Debbie is a 56-year-old living
with anorexia nervosa

The most unsupportive thing a person can do is to say how awful I look or that I'm too skinny. To a person suffering from anorexia, that is the best compliment there is. It is not the least bit helpful, and it certainly doesn't inspire me to eat or gain weight. Another unsupportive gesture is being watched. If I'm eating with another person and she is constantly watching me, whether directly or discreetly, it's a sign of distrust. My gut instinct is to stop eating immediately to regain control of the situation. I think as a general rule people are well meaning, and they believe these actions or comments are going to give me a push in the right direction. They actually invite the opposite. I think that anyone who has a friend or family member suffering from an eating disorder should get as much information and education on the subject as she can. That, I believe, is the best way to help someone. At one treatment center where I was evaluated, they gave me a folder of information not only for myself, but also to share with family and friends. The information included things NOT to say or do to a person with an eating disorder, as well as what you can do to support her. I think that would be helpful for anyone who has a family member or friend with an eating disorder.

*

DENISE PURCELL
Denise is a 50-year-old living
with anorexia nervosa and bulimia

That's an easy one: don't comment on anyone's weight, ever. They can look beautiful, but the slightest comment to someone you who is living with these demons might trigger them. It's not your fault, but it doesn't matter. It should never be about how someone looks, even though, honestly, isn't that the first thing you notice? Men and women alike have this struggle. Let's all just be us.

*

HADDI TREBISOVSKY
Haddi is a 29-year-old living
with anorexia nervosa

I certainly don't blame anyone for the things they said to me, because no one knew I was struggling. However, it wasn't helpful to hear comments about my weight or the appearance of my body. Often people would comment on how thin I was, and sometimes they said this in jealousy. These types of comments only solidified my feeling that my weight was part of my identity and I needed to protect my thinness at all costs. I also experienced a few sarcastic remarks like "Eat a burger," which were never helpful because it was only teasing and there was no real concern. If there had been concern behind the sarcasm, I never would have known it. If you feel the need to comment on someone's appearance or weight, I'd recommend taking a moment to think about why you want to say something. If you are truly concerned, think of a tactful way to bring it up. If it's merely out of jealousy, it's probably best to just keep it to yourself. As is apparent in my case, you never know what someone is struggling with, so be mindful of how you talk about sensitive topics like weight and appearance.

*

CHAPTER SEVENTEEN

Health Insurance Challenges

> Insurance - an ingenious modern game of chance in which the player is permitted to enjoy the comfortable conviction that he is beating the man who keeps the table. -AMBROSE BIERCE

Eating disorders have the highest mortality rate of any mental illness, yet finding insurance coverage to help with treatment and recovery can be challenging. What has been your experience with health insurance in relation to your recovery?

*

JUNE ALEXANDER
June is a 65-year-old living
beyond anorexia nervosa

In Australia, I pay for private health insurance. Without this, I doubt I would be alive today, because I would not have been able to afford the treatment I needed to save my life. Some of the lessons in acquiring vital health care support were tough. When I crashed and had suicidal tendencies during the breakdown of my marriage, my psychiatrist (Prof) arranged my first admission as an inpatient in a private mental health service. Several days later, when able to think a little straighter, I felt horrified to learn that my private health insurance did not cover anywhere near the full cost of the accommodation or treatment. Prof calmly pointed out the number of days until payment was due. After that, interest would accrue. "Borrow the money," he suggested. This was an early lesson in action beats anxiety. I didn't have the money to pay the bill.

Part of me felt helpless. I wanted to say that I couldn't do this (the unexpected hospital expense, on top of chronic anxiety, depression and eating disorder, seemed a punishment for being weak-minded), but something about Prof's calm and matter-of-fact manner gave me strength, made me determined. I could not ask anyone in the family for assistance, but was able to arrange a bank loan. To pay it off, I began a Saturday shift at the newspaper office. This meant working six days a week and sacrificing precious time with my children for three months. The loan was paid on time and I learned an important lesson in accepting responsibility and refusing to be a victim.

The cost of treating an eating disorder in Australia can vary greatly. The National Eating Disorders Collaboration in 2016 provides the following information.

The costs of your individual treatment will depend on what type of treatment is needed, how frequently it is needed and where the treatment is performed. It is vital to talk to clinicians, therapists and treatment professionals about the costs involved in your treatment before the treatment begins.

Medicare may cover some or all costs related to different types of eating disorder treatments. If you are hospitalized in a public hospital because you are in need of medical care Medicare may also cover some of your costs for hospital treatment.

It is important to keep in mind that there are low-cost and no-cost treatment options available for eating disorder treatments although access to them can be limited.

For further information, contact your local Medicare office or speak to your clinician or therapist about the costs involved in treatment before you commence treatment or therapy.

If you have private health insurance, you may be able to claim certain expenses that arise from treatment of your eating disorder (for example, psychology or psychiatric counseling services). What you will be able to claim and how much you will get back will depend on your specific insurance policy. In some cases, your private health insurance may not cover your expenses at all.

To find out more, you will need to obtain the relevant item number/s from your medical professionals and talk to your private healthcare provider about whether those particular service items are covered by your insurance (nedc.com.au/treatment-costs).

When you have to pay a lot of money for consultations, you may think twice about going. Unfortunately, this just gives the illness more time to embed itself in your thoughts and behaviors. Ideally, long-term support needs to be provided for people with an eating disorder. Step-down care, from inpatient clinic or hospital admissions, is vital to help avoid relapse. Going home without support is like taking a cake out of the oven when it is half-baked. You sink, you cannot cope, and you can get caught in a revolving door scenario requiring regular inpatient stays and relapsing as soon as you go home. With each failure, the illness embeds itself a little more. More home support upon leaving inpatient care is vital.

Early intervention is another crucial factor. Family doctors and clinicians need to be skilled up so they can recognize symptoms and apply early intervention treatment. This gives the best chance of full recovery and resumption of mainstream life, within weeks rather than months or years.

Families, who are usually the main caregivers, also require support and the opportunity to learn coping skills, as their homes have to double as treatment centers for the duration of the illness. Postponing a doctor's appointment because you don't have enough money to pay the bill is a sad, sad state of affairs. Postponement can add years to the duration of the illness or worse, and it may be worse than that. Families and sufferers need support. In the long run, when funding support is not forthcoming early on, the health and financial cost for the sufferer, their family and the community all mount unnecessarily.

Oh, for a magic wand.

*

OLIVIA ANTHONY
Olivia is a 44-year-old living
with anorexia nervosa and bulimia

I've had many different experiences in regard to insurance and my eating disorder. I vividly remember the day I had my first experience with insurance and trying to get help. I was twenty-one and had garbage bags hidden in my bedroom for purging. I locked my bedroom door, grabbed the phone book and went to the yellow pages. My dad had a good job, but unknown to me at the time, it didn't cover anything for mental health. No one in the family knew I was desperately sick and struggling in an abusive relationship with ED. So I went down the yellow pages columns, calling office after office, getting rejected each time. Not a single counselor took my insurance. I couldn't believe it! There I was, purging xxx times a day, and I had no coverage. I went back to school and fell deeper and deeper into my eating disorder's grasp. My binges were so severe that I couldn't stand up straight, and I worried my stomach would burst. I became desperate once again for help, so I saw a wonderful counselor on campus. After several months, though, she said that she felt like she couldn't help me enough, and referred me to the Neuroscience Clinic. I had a college health insurance plan, but after seeing a therapist and psychiatrist for a while, my psychiatrist suggested that I apply for Medicaid, since my coverage was basically used up. So I did. That was a lifesaver for me!

Years later, after having my son, and also after my brief stay in an eating disorder program in a hospital, the counselor I was referred to didn't accept Medicaid. She had a huge, generous heart, though. Luckily for me, she saw me for free for the entire time I saw her—five years! I paid her what I could, but she didn't ever charge me or make me feel less than. I saw a dietitian at that time as well, and I know that she pulled many ropes to get my twice weekly appointments with her waived—for five years. I had angels working behind the scenes for me! I tried to go into an actual eating disorder center a few times, but they didn't accept Medicaid and I didn't have the money. I felt like a worthless loser already, and then being denied access to get help made me feel even more worthless. I do feel very fortunate that I received the therapy that I did. I know that many others are ruined financially because their insurance runs out. Insurance is a misnomer!

*

CHRISTINE BASTONE
Christine is a 49-year-old living
with binge eating disorder

I haven't sought any professional help with regard to my eating disorder. So I don't have any experience with health insurance in relation to it. My experience with health insurance related to the normal everyday health issues that my family faces is that while it does help financially, it can still be very difficult to come up with the money for the co-pays for the doctor and even more for prescriptions. Not to mention that it's not easy dealing with all the red tape, and it can be quite frustrating if you need something that they don't cover.

*

LISA BRUNS
Lisa is a 52-year-old living
with binge eating disorder

Insurance paid for my gastric bypass. I'd like to have a treatment center nearby that I could attend. I still have so many unaddressed issues.

*

LYNDA CHELDELIN FELL
Lynda is a 50-year-old living
with binge eating disorder

Insurance didn't play any role in my recovery because I never sought treatment. Because of my size, I hated going to the doctor. Although binge eating disorder is now included in the Diagnostic and Statistical Manual of Mental Disorders (DSM-5), many in society don't regard binge eating as a mental illness. Further, some advocate that binge eating is an addictive behavior, yet the DSM-5 doesn't include binge eating under addiction. We're caught in the crosshairs of a clinical debate.

Dr. Stanton Peele authored an article in Psychology Today dated October 10, 2013. In his article, he opined that "Addiction is the search for emotional satisfaction—for a sense of security, a sense of being loved, even a sense of control over life. But the gratification is temporary and illusory, and the behavior results instead in greater self-disgust, reduced psychological security, and poorer coping ability. That's what all addictions have in common. There is no place where this cycle is clearer than in the case of binge eating. Binge eating points clearly to the nature of the addictive experience as a self-feeding negative relationship to an object, activity, or involvement." From my personal viewpoint, I describe myself as a food addict. I found food sobriety ten years ago, but my addiction isn't cured. Some days remain harder than others, but I've learned to manage it most of the time.

It's true that not all obese people have a binge eating disorder. And not all binge eaters are obese. Yet, it is my hope that we'll change our thinking about binge eating disorder, and advocate for the National Institutes of Health to dedicate more research dollars toward finding a cure for all forms of addiction. If a lifelong smoker develops lung cancer, does society deny them life-saving treatment because they chose to put that cigarette to their mouth? Of course not. The same principle applies to binge eating and food addiction.

*

LYDIA KENYON
Lydia is a 22-year-old living
with anorexia nervosa

I have been an outpatient throughout my recovery process, but nonetheless my insurance hasn't covered much at all. Thankfully, I have been blessed with the ability to save plenty, and I've also qualified for financial assistance through our local hospital since my income has recently decreased drastically. I haven't even tried to contact my insurance company in regard to the fact that it isn't covering much, because at this point it doesn't seem worth the hassle. I think eating disorders should be treated like any other deadly illness by the insurance companies. Yes, they are mental, but they are just as serious as cancer, and deserve to be treated as such.

*

REBEKKAH KOONS
Rebekkah is a 29-year-old living with
eating disorder not otherwise specified

My insurance was good at first about paying for my therapy sessions but it covered only a certain number of sessions, and it was a low number, about fourteen sessions. This wasn't enough for me to get any benefit out of the sessions and I had to discontinue them once my free sessions were up. I lived alone and had a limited income. I could have gotten better help if they had taken it more seriously and covered any sessions I needed.

*

RUTH PAPALAS
Ruth is a 58-year-old living
with binge eating disorder

Luckily, my health insurance covered my gastric bypass fourteen years ago. Since then, with the changes in health insurance, I've run into several issues. I sought help with a revision to the gastric bypass, but have been give the runaround at each turn. I cannot find a doctor willing to do a revision in my network. They require several expensive tests to determine my eligibility. My out-of-pocket expenses are unbelievable! Doctors don't address how your weight affects everything else (heart, lungs, diabetes, knees, feet and back). I can have surgery on any of those ailments. I can get a prescription drug for any of those issues, but no real help. I believe that is because health insurance does not cover weight loss. They do cover major health issues and some prescription drugs. Maybe that's where the real money is to be made.

*

DEBBIE PFIFFNER
Debbie is a 56-year-old living
with anorexia nervosa

When I was hospitalized at the very beginning of my eating disorder, it was the early 1980s, and there was no such thing as a treatment center for eating disorders. No doctors or therapists had any experience, and there was very little knowledge of eating disorders at that time. Therefore I was hospitalized in a medical ward for malnutrition, and that included seeing a dietitian. My insurance paid for my care as they would for any illness requiring hospitalization. After leaving the hospital, I was seen by a psychologist and a psychiatrist and my insurance paid a percentage of that care. This time around, my insurance would pay only for inpatient therapy in an accredited hospital, with doctors in the unit at all times, and an emergency room in the facility. They, like a lot of insurance companies, would not pay for bundle billing, which was the policy of all the residential treatment centers I contacted. They would only pay for medical care by a doctor, sessions with a dietitian, and sessions with a psychiatrist, psychologist or accredited therapist. With the help of the National Eating Disorders Association, we managed to find one hospital in the entire country with an eating disorders program, but it was run by registered nurses only, and my insurance denied it.

My insurance company was actually very helpful to me. I have insurance through my husband's union, so everything is done locally, and the supervisor and I became well acquainted. I have to admit that I agree with my insurance company. I think the bigger problem lies with the treatment centers themselves. They insist on "bundle billing," which means they present one bill with one amount. In that bundle they bill for such things as art therapy, horticulture therapy, yoga, massage, acupuncture and acupressure. The insurance company did not believe these were necessary to my care, and I fully agreed. The treatment centers hide these things in their bundle billing and can charge thousands of dollars a week for things that the insurance company does not believe are necessary. I have to say that I agree.

I think the bigger problem is with the treatment centers and the exorbitant amounts they are allowed to charge. I asked for and received a waiver for residential treatment at a facility near my home. The waiver granted to me would include the insurance company paying for room and board, medical care, mental health care, a dietitian, and food. The woman in charge of the program made the mistake of telling me that they were going to make me participate in all the things the insurance company wouldn't pay for, and then bury them in the bill. Since that sounded a lot like insurance fraud to me, I contacted my insurance company and they ended up pulling the waiver.

I was told by another facility that they had financial resources available, but when I went for my evaluation I found out that the financial resources were high-interest bank loans. I feel very strongly that the problem lies with the treatment centers themselves and the things they get away with, rather than with the insurance companies. That has been my experience.

*

DENISE PURCELL
Denise is a 50-year-old living
with anorexia nervosa and bulimia

When I was going to therapy for my eating disorder, it was hard to find a provider who specialized in that area. It also became out-of-pocket expenses, and they limit how much therapy you need per year, like so many visits. That should be changed. Everything is different for different cases. It shouldn't define you.

*

HADDI TREBISOVSKY
Haddi is a 29-year-old living
with anorexia nervosa

Because I didn't receive treatment specifically for my ED, I can't speak to the health insurance issue directly. However, I have received counseling as treatment for depression and anxiety (which helped in managing my ED as well), and my insurance covered it completely with a twenty-dollar copay, just like any other medical appointment. I only had to find a clinic that was listed as covered by my insurance company, and I found one that is less than ten minutes from my house. I've been very fortunate in having the coverage I've needed.

*

CHAPTER EIGHTEEN

Finding Recovery

> The road to recovery will not always be easy, but I will take it one day at a time, focusing on the moments I've dreamed about for so long.
> -AMANDA LINDHOUT

The dictionary defines recovery as a return to a normal state of health, mind, or strength. Another definition is the action or process of regaining possession or control of something stolen or lost. When looking to the future after facing an eating disorder, what does recovery mean to you?

*

JUNE ALEXANDER
June is a 65-year-old living
beyond anorexia nervosa

At my second consultation with the psychiatrist (Prof) who would save my life, he said, "You're not to give up hope. You've had the illness more than twenty years, and it will take time to get well." He had diagnosed me, at age thirty-three, with chronic anxiety and depression in addition to the eating disorder. At the time, I was full of self-doubt and was scared to hope. But Prof helped me to see that "hope" was an essential element in healing. I learned to hope, no matter what. There were many slips and slides along the way, but with Prof's guidance, I held on to hope, and it lit the path to freedom.

Recovery from an eating disorder can be like learning to ride a bicycle—at first it is wobbly, dangerous, and difficult. Taking both feet off the ground and pushing on the pedals in a bid to move forward is plain scary. Time and repeated efforts are necessary to develop a sense of trust and balance. Only when we achieve this do we start to feel safe and secure; slowly we feel confident enough to start looking around, engaging in life, and accelerating our progress. As someone who developed anorexia nervosa in 1962 and was not diagnosed for twenty years, my experience comes from the survivor end of the spectrum. I was an adult and the mother of four young children when I started to my ride to recovery.

Early intervention with the Maudsley Approach or family-based treatment (FBT) is the best solution for most children and adolescents, but many miss the opportunity for this help, and the illness becomes embedded in our identity, masterfully manipulating our thoughts and behaviors as though we were puppets on a string. Adults with eating disorders can face an enormous struggle in finding the right help to guide them to recovery. It does not help that the medical profession has differing views on which treatments work best.

When I started to seek help in the late 1970s, five or six years of misdiagnosis passed before a psychiatrist, Prof, recognized the illness and began addressing it. Prof prescribed drugs that certainly saved my life at the time, as I was chronically depressed and anxious, but they did nothing to help me understand who I was, connect me with my feelings, or challenge eating disorder behaviors and thoughts. The years rolled by; I struggled from one year to the next, my diaries full of eating disorder-fueled thoughts. My life was only a part-life at best.

Love for my children inspired my continued efforts to escape the black hole—all that was left of my soul —in which the eating disorder kept me prisoner.

By now I had been seeing Prof for fifteen years. There had to be another way out of this blackness, this helplessness, this hole. Deep down I knew that to be free, it was up to me. In an effort to provide my tortured brain with nutrition, I saw a dietitian. This dietitian did not talk about food. She talked about feelings. She helped me see which thoughts and behaviors belonged to my illness, and which belonged to the real me. This magical insight helped enormously in liberating myself from the debilitating illness. It enabled a gradual (total) rebuild of self, and development of coping skills to eliminate deeply embedded eating disorder thoughts and behaviors.

People, whether they are patients or clinicians, cannot be separated into boxes. Lines are blurred in the real world —in the home, as opposed to university research environments, hospitals and treatment centers. Yes, we need theory, we need evidence-based research, but we also need practice. We need to allow movement, to allow the research outcomes to become part of our everyday treatment options. Recovery and healing require team effort. Knowledge is no use—in fact, it is useless—unless the therapist or caretaker passionately believes the message he or she is delivering, and has skills to help the patient believe likewise, which leads to trust. Establishment of trust is essential between therapist (clinician, dietitian, and caretaker) and patient to achieve a successful outcome. The patient needs to feel safe enough to let go of his or her eating disorder thoughts and behaviors and follow guidance. My dietitian had this knack. She enabled me to feel safe and secure. She could have been a psychologist or psychiatrist, or social worker, or family-based treatment therapist. She happened to be a dietitian with training in mindfulness and FBT. She happened to be the one who connected with the tiny thread of self that remained within my soul.

Regarding food amounts/nutrition in early stages of recovery, it is like learning to ride a bicycle. Little kids use training wheels. The wheels give them security and stability until they get their confidence up. When they let the trainer wheels go, they excitedly find they have more freedom and can go faster, they can go anywhere they like. Set amounts of food also can give security and stability, until the patient gets his or her confidence up, and can start letting go of set foods, set amounts, set routines, set behaviors and thought patterns, set life. It is a gradual process. This is how it was for me—a chronic, long-term anorexia/bulimia sufferer, now free of eating disorder behaviors. It doesn't matter how old the kid is when they get on that bike. If it has training wheels, if they have a trustworthy guide who believes in them, the kid can learn, build confidence, throw away the training wheels and embrace freedom.

For children and adolescents where early intervention is possible, implementation of family-based treatment can quickly get them back on the road of life, but for the person who has missed early intervention, and the eating disorder is embedded, the assistance of a dietitian and other health practitioners on the treatment team can be helpful.

The good thing about family-based treatment is that ideally, it involves all members of the family. This is important because an eating disorder affects all members of a family. Recovery without family support is tough. But it can be achieved with the support of at least one person in whom trust is established. The most important factor in any recovery guide, whatever their profession is, simply, trust. When we trust, we can ride our bike anywhere. See more at www.nationaleatingdisorders.org.

My story adds to the evidence that recovery can be achieved at any age. And what is recovery, anyway? I prefer the word *freedom*; freedom to eat what I want, when I want, without feeling shame, stigma or guilt (sugar on my rhubarb makes it taste so much better); freedom to wear clothes I want, to take part in activities I want, go places I want, without feeling shame, stigma or guilt. This is what I call recovery. I'll never know if I am the person I would have been if I had not developed anorexia nervosa at age eleven. What I do know is that at age sixty-five, I am free. My silver lining is the freedom to embrace the beauty of each day, to enjoy my family and friends, to help others however I can, and to be a best friend to myself. This is my silver lining.

Another thing I know for sure: There is hope at every age. I can hardly believe I am the same person who lived in the darkness of an eating disorder for four decades, but I know I am, and this makes life more beautiful.

Rolling up my sleeve, in 2013, and donating a blood sample for gene research and discovery was one of the most meaningful moments in my life. My blood sample, along with many others, was collected as part of the Anorexia Nervosa Genetics Initiative, a global effort to identify genes that contribute to eating disorders. To know that I am contributing in a small way to helping researchers find a cure for anorexia nervosa feels good. Really, really good. The opportunity to contribute to science and help find a cure for the illness that tormented and almost took my life was emotionally overwhelming. Half a century after I developed anorexia nervosa, there I was, giving a blood sample to help find out why.

I cried tears in my soul that day. Tears for my parents who were not alive to know about this research. Tears especially for my mother, because she did not understand what happened to her younger daughter, me, at age eleven. She didn't understand that I had an illness in my brain. She certainly did not know that part of the reason was genetic. She did not know how to help me. She did not know the real me was suppressed by this illness; she did not know that the little girl she knew but had disappeared was imprisoned deep inside, crying and trying to get out. It was so difficult, without a guide to help her, or me.

As the years rolled by, misunderstandings became mountains that could not be crossed. I became alienated from my mother and father and my sister. Anorexia nervosa affects the sufferer most, but also affects, in some way, every member of the family.

It affected my marriage, too. When I walked down the aisle at age twenty to marry George, my childhood sweetheart, anorexia nervosa went with me. I could not shake it off. It was worse than a monkey on my back.

It was a black octopus in my brain. Eventually it destroyed my marriage. My love of writing and love for my children helped me survive, and eventually, in my thirties, I began to meet health professionals who understood the illness and set me on the long road to recovery. I had felt lost in a dark forest for decades; now I was receiving help to find a way out—and regain me. At age fifty-five, I gained my freedom from anorexia nervosa and began writing books to help others who, through no fault of their own, were suffering this illness. Helping others has been the most meaningful and fulfilling way to make my life, and my suffering and loss, count. So I have found, and continue to find, many silver linings, including the opportunity to contribute to the Real Life Diaries!

*

OLIVIA ANTHONY
Olivia is a 44-year-old living
with anorexia nervosa and bulimia

Recovery. With my marriage to ED, I've had a lifetime with our relationship being on-again, off-again. So in the past, during each reprieve from suffering in that mental prison, I thought I had conquered ED, that I had kicked him to the curb, that I had gotten the big D from him. Then I relapsed and felt like a failure again for succumbing to his sweet nothings. Argh. I look at my life now and again believe that I have ended my relationship with ED. This time I have more hope that ED won't ever move back into my head. I've healed a lot of false beliefs that I had had about myself, and have healed a lot of pain that I had held inside for so long. I don't use food or the restriction of food as a mood-altering drug any longer. I love food and I also love being strong. Recovery for me is about honoring myself. I'm still learning, but I'm so much better at stating my needs or opinions. If something upsets me, I talk about it eight times out of ten. That's a lot better than before. In the past it was my pattern to keep quiet, and then either restrict food or eat and then purge. A big part of recovery for me is accepting my body no matter what. Not comparing myself to others is also a big part of my staying healthy. That one is hard to do! But, it gets easier each day I do it. For that I am grateful.

In my dysfunctional relationship with ED, I definitely have learned to have more empathy for others. I love talking to people and finding out what their lives have been like. I really want to help others in some way. I always have, but with ED as part of my history, I know that I will have much more to offer. I know what it's like to feel like life is pointless and I'm a huge waste of space. I've attempted suicide. I've truly been to the bottom of the barrel. Had I not experienced that, I wouldn't be who I am today. I really hope to be of service.

*

CHRISTINE BASTONE
Christine is a 49-year-old living
with binge eating disorder

Recovery would mean that I was at a normal weight. Recovery would mean that I ate a normal quantity of food. Recovery would mean that food was of normal importance. Recovery would mean that I was comfortable in my clothes, and that I didn't have to constantly pull my shirt down. Recovery would mean that I never, or at least very rarely, binged. Recovery would mean that I ate only three normal meals a day, with no more than a snack or two in addition to that. Recovery would mean that I could eat at a buffet and be full, but not stuffed when I was done. Recovery would mean that most of the time I eat only when physically hungry, and would meet my emotional needs and hungers in other ways.

Recovery would mean I didn't feel like an bottomless empty pit that I needed to try to fill up with food. That is what recovery means to me, and at this point it feels like a very beautiful but impossible dream.

*

LISA BRUNS
Lisa is a 52-year-old living
with binge eating disorder

I feel like I should be grateful that I was able to have gastric bypass. I see people who are larger than me, but I always feel like I'm the elephant in the room.

*

LYNDA CHELDELIN FELL
Lynda is a 50-year-old living
with binge eating disorder

My brother is an alcoholic, and we have discussed the similarities between our challenges many times. Recovery to me would mean finding a cure for not just binge eating, but for addictions of all kinds. Offering medication and surgical options for binge eating don't solve the underlying illness. Why is a cure out of the realm of possibility? It would reduce the high demand placed on our healthcare industry from comorbidities that stem from obesity. Recovery to me would mean a cure of some type so the burden of addiction could be lifted.

*

LYDIA KENYON
Lydia is a 22-year-old living
with anorexia nervosa

Recovery means freedom. I no longer feel trapped by my own mind. I feel like I can socialize more, and eat much more freely. Not only does my health now mean a lot to me, but I know it has always meant a lot to my family. I'm so happy to be able to make them, and myself, proud. For so long, I thought I could put myself in their shoes. I felt so heartbroken for them, and anyone else who was dealing with any form of mental illness, but I had no compassion for myself. Finding self-worth has been an ongoing battle, but I feel like I am getting there, step by step.

*

REBEKKAH KOONS
Rebekkah is a 29-year-old living with
an eating disorder not otherwise specified

Recovery to me means hope. It means I've gotten through the hardest part medically but now have to tackle the emotionally hard parts, but it means I have hope.

*

RUTH PAPALAS
Ruth is a 58-year-old living
with binge eating disorder

If I could see recovery, it would start by weighing what my driver's license says I weigh. After the gastric bypass, I was ecstatic to go and get a new driver's license with a much, much lower weight. As my weight crept back up, I withheld my hope that it was only temporary and I would eventually (sooner rather than later) go back to that weight. I'm still hopeful and still waiting. Recovery would look like I was finally happy and confident in my own skin and that I have achieved a body that looks good. It would mean I could get rid of three sizes of clothes (some are smaller, just in case, and some are larger, also just in case) and keep only the ones that fit in that perfect size. It would mean that I wouldn't have to try on six different things to find out which outfit is not going to highlight my size. I literally own hundreds of clothing items, hundreds! And yet I have nothing to wear.

It would mean that I would eat for actual hunger and nutrition only and not to reward myself for getting through a rough day. Food would not be a treat because I had a good day and I'm celebrating! It would mean that I've finally wrapped my head and my mouth around the fact that food is needed only for nutrition and not just pleasure.

Recovery would mean I could stop my tendency to turn to food in response to emotional issues. It would mean that I could wake up and not even have to think "This is the day…" because I wouldn't even have to think about it. I would wake up as the perfect me instead of waking up to find out I'm still me, and still weigh this much. Recovery seems more like a dream than a reality.

*

DEBBIE PFIFFNER
Debbie is a 56-year-old living
with anorexia nervosa

My eating disorder has redefined my life in ways that I could never have imagined as a teenager, intent on getting as thin as I possibly could. I suffer on a daily basis, both physically and emotionally. I have not seen, nor do I believe I ever will see a silver lining to all this. The fact that after being in recovery for many years and thinking it could never happen again, but I ended up right back where I started from, confirms that this will always be an issue for me. I may be in recovery at this time, but I will never be over it and it will always be a struggle.

*

DENISE PURCELL
Denise is a 50-year-old living
with anorexia nervosa and bulimia

While I know why I have this problem, it's an everyday battle with my mind. It's control versus not feeling in control. While I wasn't able to cure myself, I did learn enough to teach my girls that eating disorders are real and stem from a lot of different reasons. But they are beautiful. It's not up to anyone to determine who you should be or what you should look like. But the struggle is real, and no one has to feel alone when dealing with it.

*

HADDI TREBISOVSKY
Haddi is a 29-year-old living
with anorexia nervosa

I have always believed that everything happens for a reason, or at least there can always be something to be learned from an experience. Those years of struggle did indeed have their place in defining who I am today, and fortunately I can say that with gratification.

Growing up, I was very insecure and had very low self-esteem. In many ways this was why I began skipping meals. For several years my image was what defined me, and I kept that definition consistent through my eating disorder. Because of my struggle, I was forced to come face to face with my issues and I had a choice to either ignore them, knowing that I could never get better that way, or confront them, which is what I ultimately chose. Choosing recovery was not easy. I had been very comfortable in my coping mechanisms, even though they were incredibly unhealthy, and the thought of breaking free from them was overwhelming and exhausting and sounded impossible. Ever since I chose recovery, decisions around my health have become increasingly easier.

Even though I still struggle sometimes (currently I'm six weeks postpartum and my hormones are all over the place), there have certainly been days when I feel overwhelmed, hopeless, and depressed. I say this to let you know that even though I consider myself recovered, difficulties still happen, I've learned what warning signs to look out for and I'm able to make decisions over my mental health with less and less guilt. Since choosing recovery years ago, I believe I'm in a good place so that I can help others. In fact, I think that's the biggest way my eating disorder has redefined my life: because I've lived through an eating disorder, I can be there for others who are having a hard time right now. My experience has value in helping others feel less alone, less isolated, less of an outcast for dealing with the things they are dealing with. My sincere hope in sharing my story in this book is that someone will feel encouraged and will even find recovery for themselves because of what they read about my life. For me, that would absolutely be a silver lining to having an eating disorder!

*

walking the Journey

Be like the birds, sing after every storm.
-BETH MENDE CONNY

Every journey is as unique as one's fingerprint, for we experience different beliefs, different desires, different needs, different tolerances, and often we walk different roads. Though we might not see anyone else on the path, we are never truly alone, for more walk behind, beside, and in front of us. In this chapter lies the answers to the final question posed: What would you like the world to know about your eating disorder journey?

*

JUNE ALEXANDER
June is a 65-year-old living
beyond anorexia nervosa

I would like the world to know that at every age, it is possible to heal from an eating disorder. Not only heal, but live a full and productive life. Often, the traits that have been self-destructing when aligned with the eating disorder, become powerful self-construction traits when aligned with true self. The importance of family and friends in recovery and relapse prevention is explored in the following blog www.junealexander.com, in November 2015.

Families and friends, where does one start and the other end? For me, there is no beginning and no end. I reflect and marvel at how, at any age, new growth can bud. Family and friends encircle me. Their many elements form a priceless ring of love and support. When I waver, I am encouraged back on track; I'm told "You can do it," "Try again," when I admit I've failed again. The people who form my ring have endless quantities of patience and understanding, unconditional faith, and acceptance. For I am a challenge. The people who form my ring are my life raft; they keep me afloat. Some have been there forever, others more recently and, like rings on a tree, they all have a role, and are a part of me.

Childhood: Parents, sister, grandparents; cousins, aunts and uncles, school friends. Until age eleven, when I developed anorexia, life was relatively uncomplicated. Adventurous-spirited and shy, a child who loved to read books and write, and wanted everyone to be happy. My story is told in my memoir, *A Girl Called Tim*. Childhood is a defining period; it sets much of the pattern on how to handle what comes next. Children are like flowers. We bud and burst into bloom, we blossom, fully or partially, and only time will tell. Creation itself is a miracle, with traits inherited, genetic template fixed. When one is born with a vulnerability for an eating disorder, many factors come into play. The illness may be obvious or obscure, hidden in layers of secrets, as mine was for decades. Sadly, as a result of my eating disorder, and related factors, I became isolated from many people who were dear to me. Throughout, however, my diary has been a confidante, and a survival tool (unknowingly, at times, also a self-destructive tool) since age eleven.

Adolescence: My anorexia, untreated, morphed into bulimia-anorexia in my teenage years, so I looked normal even though I did not feel it. I did not know it then, but I know now, that the sneaky illness thoroughly took over my mind. Sabotaged it. Caused me to think and behave in ways that were not true to me. My mother asked and pleaded: Why can't you be like (friend) and (friend)? I wanted to be. I just didn't know how. Part of my true self was disintegrating under the force of the illness. But some good things were happening, too. I tried to cope by doing well at school and creating a sense of belonging where I could, which was mostly with my best friend Helen. At age sixteen, I met George, who would become my husband four years on, and I became an American Field Service exchange student to Missouri, USA, for a year. My host family, the Edwards, remain my second family. A passion for writing led to a cadetship with a country newspaper at age eighteen, and so began a career in journalism.

Twenties and Thirties: Good times and bad times. Married at twenty, but manipulative ED came too. Eight weeks later my car collided with a log truck on my way to work, causing cervical spine injuries, the effects of which continue today. Four beautiful children by the age of twenty-five. Then the anxiety and depression that had been building since childhood, led to suicidal thoughts. At age twenty-seven, love of my husband and four children gave me strength to seek help for the first time and share my story with a general practitioner. Six years of misdiagnosis ensued, eventually leading me to Professor Graham Burrows, who became my psychiatrist for the next thirty years. He saved my life but there was a cost. I lost my husband and my family of origin. Such can be the effects of a long-term eating disorder. I loved them all but behaved as if I didn't. Reading my diaries from this time is difficult, for I am so not me. My many rules and lists for getting through each day, and inevitably failing, played right into ED's scheming ways. I was on a roundabout, spiraling downward into a deep dark well. Thank goodness the family and friendship circle enveloping me at that time was sufficiently strong to keep alive a thread within that said "I want to be free." I wanted to show that I could be true to the real 'me'. I am here, just almost buried in layers of isolation, crying within and trying to escape this non-stop hell.

Forties: Good things happen. My family-friend circle grows. Strange things may happen when you have an eating disorder for a long time. I learned at an early age not to talk to my family of origin about the eating disorder or inner feelings and thoughts. Mental health challenges were considered a sign of weakness and inability to cope; safe topics were preferred, like talking about the weather or politics or the price of food or fuel, or what others were doing. In this way, my family-friendship ring began to develop a divergence. Alienation from my family of origin began, a painful process; luckily, however, at the same time a strengthening began to evolve. Increasingly, in striving to reconnect my body with lost self, I developed sufficient trust to start sharing long suppressed thoughts and feelings with my psychiatrist, minister of religion, best friends. Whether or not they understood, they tolerated and accepted me, assured me that fresh starts were good, that failures were opportunities for learning when lost to the eating disorder. Two more important people became fresh components of my life ring—Belinda, who taught me about mindfulness, and a general practitioner who remains a caring guide until this day. My diary began to become a source of self-help rather than self-destruction.

Fifties: A wonderful decade. After forty-four years of living under ED's rules, bullying and torment, I break free. Free to discover and develop my true identity. Many people to thank. Especially my lifeblood, my now adult children, forever supportive and loving, accepting and tolerating, if not understanding, their mother's many sideways steps; and their dad, an ever-reliable anchor when storms hit, a few words is often all it takes, in guiding me to shore. It was this family, my family of choice, together with health professionals, who helped me cross the line to me. And a new little cheer squad began to form with the birth of my first grandchild. This support gave me strength to let my inner self step into the light, start sharing my story publicly, and this sharing brought fresh revelations: first, the release of my memoir, *A Girl Called Tim*, and *My Kid is Back* led to the overwhelming discovery that there are many others who have suffered, are suffering, like me. Friends and family, they are one.

Moreover, the release of these books, and others, on eating disorders led to the creation of another kind of family, a global family with whom I feel safe, supported and secure. This is my family in the eating disorder field. I can share thoughts and feelings with this family. How amazing is this? Goodbye to shame and stigma. Goodbye to pretense. Hello to being me. My body and self are one. Hello to acceptance and enriching self-belief. I'm so glad I persevered and did not give up.

Sixties: I am supposed to be old and wise by now, but many parts of me remain young, exploring and catching up on experiences and growth that were sabotaged for decades by the eating disorder. I continue to make mistakes, the sort that were missed during adolescence and young adulthood due to the eating disorder's disintegration of self. Food is my daily medicine, but recovery from an eating disorder involves far more than this. For me, intimate, interpersonal relationships remain a challenge: to accept that it is okay, a right for me as for all, to live in an environment that is safe, secure and stable. My children seem so wise; they accept me, with my imperfections; as they have grown into fine young adults, two becoming parents themselves, they have taken on the roles of patient guides, mentors and carers. Each provides support in his or her own way. Lucky me. Longtime friends do the same, and in the eating disorder field, my other family continues to grow and grow. The internet and social media facilitate connecting and developing a sense of belonging.

Friendships continue to develop with each new year, with totally amazing people, some in person, and others solely online. They range from people with an eating disorder to emeritus professors, whose acceptance has led to the writing of more books and advocacy in the eating disorder field. In giving, one receives.

Helping others helps heal oneself. These are my lessons. If you are facing a challenge, persevere, for the storm will pass and the sun will shine again. Reaching out, seeking help, will help the clouds pass by that much sooner.

The new generations: Researchers tell us that there is quite a strong genetic component in people who develop eating disorders, and this subject is close to my heart. When I was a child there was no awareness of signs or symptoms of an eating disorder, let alone any genetic vulnerability, and my parents and the doctors had no idea how to help me. Today, however, we can arm ourselves with knowledge and, if feeling at all concerned, seek early intervention.

With this in mind, I penned the following letters to my eldest granddaughter, Olivia Rose, who was born December 23, 2009.

December 27, 2009

Dear Olivia Rose,

Right now you are a sweet wee babe wrapped snug in a rug and bunny suit. By the time you are old enough to read this letter, I picture you as a happy, bubbly little girl hopping from one foot to the other without a care in the world.

Olivia Rose, I will be forever telling you that you are very special and very loved. This is not because you are my first granddaughter, or because you were born on your great-grandmother Anne's birthday, but because you are you.

I cuddled and kissed you when you were a few hours old. You were sound asleep and yet already radiated serenity and self-assurance. Somehow you indicated you are aware of your role in life, and that as you grow up you will quietly and confidently go about fulfilling it. I am sure I felt this as I held you, Olivia Rose. I didn't only wish it. My heart was filled with gladness.

When I was a little girl, I felt confused and unsure of myself. I enjoyed going to school, and did my best to get top marks but felt upset and cross with myself when I made a mistake. Then, at age eleven, an event occurred which made me feel very anxious. I felt alone and scared, Olivia Rose, and an illness called anorexia nervosa developed in my brain. Basically, I felt afraid to eat. My mum and dad did not know what to do, because back then there was no family-based treatment like there is now.

Untreated, my anorexia set in and took over my thoughts. When I was a teenager, it evolved into bulimia, which meant I sometimes ate a lot and other times ate nothing. I felt very mixed up. I worried about little things and often felt sad. All up, I took forty-five years to get on top of this sneaky bunch of thoughts that were not really me, playing havoc in my brain. I'm sure you agree this is a very long time to be bossed around but the important thing is that now I am free, Olivia Rose.

With much help from doctors and loving support from your Grandpa George, your mum Amanda and Uncles Shane, Rohan and Ben, I have picked up the threads of my childhood, and am having great fun catching up on living my life. You will see!

I have been free for four years now and keep healthy by taking care of my feelings as they arise—reaching out for help if I need to —and eating three meals and three snacks a day. I feel like a bird soaring and swooping with glee in the clear sunny sky—such is my joy on escaping the darkness that was my illness.

When I started my recovery journey, I had to work out what thoughts belonged to me, and what thoughts belonged to my illness. I had to be brave enough to trust the thoughts that belonged to me and push the other thoughts away. I liken this process to that of a small bird with weak wings, flying for the first time. I dropped to the ground more than a few times but amazingly my thoughts got stronger as I persevered and gradually learned to trust myself and others. Now that my wings and sense of self are strong I am devoted to giving hope to others. I am flying around the world with this message.

My wish is for you and other children to grow up feeling happy and confident, free to achieve your dreams and live your life to the full.

Olivia Rose, I am glad I did not give up, that I reached out and found help to beat my illness, because I am here to enjoy you and our beautiful family. If you ever feel a worry coming on, remember that we are here to listen and to help. And you might as well get used to it now—as your grandma I will be forever reminding you that to soar like a bird, you must simply eat three meals and three snacks every day!

Love always, Grandma June

May 27, 2015

Dear Olivia Rose,

Already you are five years old. You are a bubbly and sweet little girl who indeed does not only hop a lot, but also does cartwheels, hangs upside over my bedside and says with glee: "Grandma, I absolutely love gymnastics." When I take you to school on my weekly grandma day, you happily say goodbye and run to join the morning lineup for Prep Class. You love art, rainbows and colors, jigsaw puzzles, reading and writing; you go swimming and play golf, and oh, how you love to run. You manage admirably to define you, placed as you are, between big brother Lachlan and little sister Amelia. You understand that to do all the activities you love, to the best of your ability, that your body needs nourishment with regular, nutritious meals and snacks. You are indeed soaring like a bird through life and watching you embrace such freedom makes my heart sing.

I am ever grateful that I persevered in recovering from the eating disorder that developed in my brain, causing disintegration of self, when I was a little girl. It was hard work, reconnecting with myself, but nine years into recovery, relapse prevention is easy, because I have the best medicine in the world: I have you. Family love and acceptance has a special power and strength that doctors cannot prescribe.

Olivia Rose, since my previous letter, I have begun a Ph.D. in Creative Writing related to my illness experience, and am writing several more books about eating disorders. Every time you visit, you find me at my laptop, writing. You sit beside me and engage in your own quiet pursuit. Already you are saying, "I want to be a doctor when I grow up, like Grandma." With such a comment, there is only one thing for me to do in this, my sixty-fifth year, and that is to keep writing, keep eating three meals and three snacks a day.

We are a team, for sure. We have no secrets. If ever signs or symptoms of "ED" appear, we will recognize them, talk and pounce on them, quickly.

The reason I continue to write, and go to conferences, and advocate about eating disorders, is because we still don't know what causes them. We need more research, and for more research we need more funding. This is why I am sharing our story in eating disorder awareness campaigns.

I hope, in your lifetime Olivia Rose, that we will know what causes an eating disorder, and that children everywhere will be able to grow up in a supportive environment, both within families and in accessing health services that provide evidence-based care.

Love always, Grandma June

The benefits of letter writing as a self-healing and therapeutic tool are explored in *Using Writing as a Therapy for Eating Disorders - The Diary Healer* (http://bit.ly/24IOF5S).

If you suspect symptoms of an eating disorder, early intervention with evidence-based treatment offers the best prognosis and the best chance to quickly resume living your life to the full. However, if this early opportunity for intervention has been missed, and you have been experiencing eating disorder symptoms for years, hold onto hope. Explore the online resources listed on page ix, and ask your local doctor for a referral to a specialist with eating disorder expertise. My take home message is that healing from an eating disorder is possible at every age. The first step is to reach out for help.

*

OLIVIA ANTHONY
Olivia is a 44-year-old living
with anorexia nervosa and bulimia

I've had an on-again, off-again relationship with ED. During the years when I kicked ED out, I thought I was done with him. I thought he would never return. I've worked with many different therapists through the decades. The last time I relapsed, I was really hard on myself because I was forty and I had beat it, or so I thought. The therapist I had at the time helped me to see that each time I struggled with my eating disorder, I was peeling back another layer of myself that was ready to be healed. Also, the doctor who said, "When are you going to stop that adolescent behavior?" stuck in my head all that time. Eating disorders are not an adolescent issue! Sure, adolescents suffer from eating disorders, but eating disorders are not just an adolescent issue. Just as drugs like heroin and meth aren't adolescent issues, neither is the coping mechanism of eating disorders. So dropping shame from that helped me, too.

This last time I relapsed, I saw that I really can't ever depend on ED being there for me. Oh, sure, he'll gladly be waiting for me with a dozen roses in hand if I decide to let him in. But I learned that I cannot depend on it. Interestingly, toward the end of my letting my eating disorder call the shots during that last relapse, it stopped working for me. When I purged, it wasn't a great release of endorphins like it used to be. I'm grateful for that now. My body has been through so much. I don't know how I lived through it.

I do believe that I reached so far into myself to the core of my reasons for reaching out to it that I won't fall for the urge for sweet nothings again. With hypnosis as part of my toolbox this last time, I really learned that I'm not a horrible person. I had some difficult and horrible things done to me, but I'm no victim. I believe that I changed my beliefs about myself through hypnosis, and that will help me say NO to ED if he ever chooses to ask me back. And I do admit that with this baby weight to lose, and with the relationship changes that naturally occurred due to having a new baby with my sweet hubby, I have had fleeting thoughts about how easy (see the smooth talker that ED is??) it would be to just get rid of the xxx I ate. But then I looked at myself in the mirror with my beautiful baby and looked at my body, and I thought about how happy I was to find that dead-end sign on the street that ED lives on. It is a dead end to embrace ED.

Part of my journey has been to love myself, to love my body, no matter what. That's tough to do! My daughter is so beautiful in her delightfully chubby body. I don't want her to grow up to believe that she has to be thin to be beautiful. I've talked to my hubby about my desire to never talk about my body parts, especially in front of our daughter. I also don't want us to discuss other people's bodies. I don't want us to talk about our daughter's body either. I don't want her to ever look at her body and think that it should be smaller, thinner, stronger, etc. I am doing my best to thank my body for keeping me alive, for being my vehicle that allows me to live here on Earth. It's been a long road getting to this gratitude, but I know that a full recovery is possible.

*

CHRISTINE BASTONE
Christine is a 49-year-old living
with binge eating disorder

I would like the world to know that I am addicted to food, and that living with binge eating disorder is really tough. While I have no desire to minimize other addictions, the hard part about being a binge eater and food addict is that there is no getting away from food. It is everywhere. Not only is it in my house and almost everywhere I go, but I can't drive down the street without passing a restaurant. I can't watch TV without seeing food in a commercial or the characters eating being part of the program. I can't even read a book that doesn't have the characters eating, or food being mentioned or described. Not only is it everywhere, but you have to eat. I don't have to smoke, I don't have to drink alcohol, I don't have to gamble and I don't have to abuse any type of drugs...but I do have to eat. That is the unique part of food addiction.

It's terrible to almost always feel this emptiness inside. This endless and bottomless pit that I am always trying to fill up with food. While my physical hunger is big, my emotional hunger is intense. It is also constant, unless I am completely full or even stuffed. And even then it will be back in only a few hours.

Binges don't have to be followed by vomiting to be a problem. And as I have recently learned, eating disorders are not always the anorexia and bulimia that we typically think of when we hear the words "eating disorder." I don't need your harsh judgment; that will only lead me to the refrigerator. But all emotions drive me to eat, happy or sad. Some people don't eat when they get really upset. I envy those people. I eat even more when I'm upset. When my sister died, my appetite was reduced for a period of time. I was disappointed that it lasted only a few weeks. I'm even more disappointed that I've wanted to eat everything in sight ever since.

Unless you are pregnant and wearing maternity clothes, clothes are not made for anyone with a big belly! Shirts ride up, pants and shorts ride down. I am constantly pulling at my clothes, trying to keep everything covered, especially my belly. It is so uncomfortable. It is also humiliating. I hate trying to decide what to wear. I hate even more going out in public. If I can stay in my car like I could when I took my kids to school, or now when I pick up my son at the bus stop...that is not too bad. But when I have to get out of the car, I dread it. And a big part of why I dread it is my clothes that I have to constantly pull at to keep the results of my bingeing covered up as much as possible. As I said earlier, I am not addicted to drugs or cigarettes or gambling or alcohol—I am addicted to food. Now, please don't think that I'm saying that other addictions are easy; I'm sure they are not. I'm only saying that binge eating and food addiction are a bit different.

Here is my experience with those other things I just mentioned: I used to be a light smoker. I mostly smoked to stay awake at work. But I stopped cold turkey on New Year's 1999 because I knew I was going to try to get pregnant that year. Occasionally I do want one, especially if I see someone else having one. But it hasn't been a big deal to resist.

When I was on my honeymoon, I played the slot machines. But I just couldn't keep putting quarters in the machine! Maybe I'm just cheap with money, but there was absolutely no way that I was going to lose any more money than the thirty dollars or so that I had set aside for gambling. I'm also a social drinker. But while I have been tipsy a time or two, I have never been drunk. I have absolutely no desire to get drunk, mostly because I want to avoid the hangover the next day. Not only that, but it's very rare that I have more than one drink.

That's not to say that I'm better than anyone who is addicted to any of those things. I'm just not tempted by those things. It's food that tempts me instead. That seemingly innocent stuff that we all have to ingest to survive. And while I might not currently have any strength against that temptation, I do plan to dwell on my answer to what recovery means to me, because it makes me feel good, and paints a beautiful picture in my head.

*

LISA BRUNS
Lisa is a 52-year-old living
with binge eating disorder

The world should know my eating disorder is very painful for me. It has defined my life. I had missed opportunities and missed a lot if life. I'm not close to my family and I don't have friends. It's very sad to me.

*

LYNDA CHELDELIN FELL
Lynda is a 50-year-old living
with binge eating disorder

I would like the world to know that binge eating is a powerful and destructive illness. It isn't a result of gluttonous or lazy behavior. It holds power over our lives, and sometimes I'm not strong enough to fight back. Eating disorders deserve more funding for research and a cure. The damage is staggering, costing millions of dollars. It also destroys relationships, careers, and entire families. Regardless of whether one views binge eating as a mental illness or addiction, I find it's shameful that our government is willing to spend millions of dollars fighting diseases in third world countries, yet ignores a growing epidemic in its own backyard.

No child ever says they want to grow up to be fat. Nobody enjoys being obese. Binge eating is a disorder we are powerless against, and few find freedom from its grip. It's up to our generation to change that.

*

LYDIA KENYON
Lydia is a 22-year-old living
with anorexia nervosa

An eating disorder isn't something you strive for. Or usually that isn't the case. I didn't even know what anorexia was before I was diagnosed with it. That right there is solid proof that an eating disorder isn't an end goal. It isn't a diet. It isn't a picture of health. An eating disorder is death knocking on your door, and a grave being dug. It's your brain turning against you. It is unintentional. I am not my eating disorder, and I never will be.

*

REBEKKAH KOONS
Rebekkah is a 29-year-old living with an
eating disorder not otherwise specified

It's not black and white. You can be a normal weight and struggle just as much as someone who is deathly thin.

*

RUTH PAPALAS
Ruth is a 58-year-old living
with binge eating disorder

Over the years I've gained and lost hundreds of pounds. There could be another whole me (or two or even more) if I hadn't lost some. I have successfully lost weight on diets and also when I had the gastric bypass. Losing weight is not the issue. Keeping it off is. I'm not at the ideal weight now, whatever that is. I'm fifty-eight years old and might never reach an ideal weight—ever.

I turn eating into a response to emotional issues. I can't stop myself once I start, and at times I can't resist starting in the first place. Food to me is both a comfort and a curse. It brings a sense of relief and satisfaction, and then self-loathing, disgust and shame. Emotional eating is hard for me, because I'm always feeling some type of emotion. It is also hard because I have to eat to live. Participation is necessary in other addictions, but food is a necessity. I have always envied people who can't eat when they are stressed, because I overeat when I'm stressed. When the feel-good part of eating subsides, guilt and self-deprecation take over. I know I've sabotaged myself again. I'm disgusted and out of control. Then it starts all over again. Tomorrow, tomorrow. I'll be good tomorrow....it's only a day away....

I know that what I'm doing is not right or normal. But it hadn't occurred to me that I had an eating disorder. I thought I had a weight problem. The hardest reality for me is that I'm the only one who can fix this or learn to live with it.

It was more difficult to participate in this book than anything else I've ever written. I'm really not a sad or depressed person. I'm a good person regardless of my size. I mean no one any harm or ill will. I love to laugh and have fun and I do both quite often. I'm actually quite positive about most things. My motto is "Every little thing is gonna be all right." The subject of weight is probably the most disturbing part of my whole life. It is hard for me to believe that I just shared as much of my weight issue/eating disorder with you as I did. It's hard to believe I even used my real name and gave permission to have a full-length picture of myself in a swimsuit in this book, but it is what it is.

Because my dream is to someday reach my ideal weight, I'll close with a quote that I need to take to heart. "Never give up on a dream because of the time it will take to accomplish it; the time will pass anyway." – Earl Nightingale

*

DEBBIE PFIFFNER
Debbie is a 56-year-old living
with anorexia nervosa

Once you have had an eating disorder, you will always think of food and eating differently than the average person does. You will always have a love/hate relationship with food and eating. My eating disorder, anorexia nervosa, has been a part of my life since the age of seventeen, and it always will be. I was in recovery for many years. My therapist would ask me every so often how I was doing with my eating disorder. I remember telling him that he didn't have to worry, that I didn't think I could ever possibly go back to not eating. And here I am today, years later, recovering yet again. When I reach my goal weight, it will not be over. It is a lifelong struggle, and I must remain aware. Just as I am an alcoholic who has been in recovery for thirteen years, I have to take one day at a time and remain vigilant. Recovery from my eating disorder will be the same —one day at time, remaining vigilant. I will never be cured. I will remain in recovery. I chose to coauthor this book and share my story so when someone who is suffering from an eating disorder and is feeling alone, they will know they are not. There is hope. There are people out there who have gone through it and would be happy to help you on your journey. You are not weak, you are ill. And remember, we are all in this together.

*

DENISE PURCELL
Denise is a 50-year-old living
with anorexia nervosa and bulimia

I would like people to know that until we stop comparing ourselves and others to people in magazines, on television, and one another, it will never end. We need to accept ourselves and one another for who we are, not what we look like or a scale number. Just because you're skinny doesn't mean you are healthy. It's not done for attention. It's real and painful and starts with a few negative words. Let's be more sensitive to the struggles of others.

*

HADDI TREBISOVSKY
Haddi is a 29-year-old living
with anorexia nervosa

About a year ago I pondered this same question because there was something bothering me whenever I heard "I will always struggle with xyz (ED, addiction, depression, etc.)." And then I understood why it irritated me. I wrote a blog post explaining those frustrations and I used my own anorexia as an example. I think the best way to convey what I'd like the world to know about my eating disorder is if I simply share an excerpt from that blog post here.

Since I've recovered I've heard and seen many people claim that having an eating disorder is a daily struggle even after recovery, and that it is something you will always battle with. I'm writing this now to present my two cents on the matter, because it finally clicked for me why this is a dangerous way to view recovery.

I am not struggling daily with my ED.

It might only come down to semantics, but this is why I can't bring myself to say that depression, ED, anxiety, and whatever else I need to recover from will always be my battle.

When we tell ourselves and others that (insert issue here) will always be a struggle, we're creating a safety net built from a pre-approved excuse for a relapse. We're taking away our power and giving it to the disorder/addiction/etc., claiming that we will never be free from it. We're also feeding into an attitude of fear. How disheartening to go through a recovery program or treatment when you've fought tooth and nail to acquire health, only to hear that you're not done fighting, and you never will be. If you become tired in battle, that only means your disorder or addiction is going to get the best of you at some point, because you and the issue are always struggling. *So if the Son sets you free, you are truly free* (John 8:36).

I think a healthier way to respond to questions or uncertainties about our recovery is to say or know for ourselves that (insert issue here) is something we are aware that we have been prone to struggle with or fall for, which is why we now x, y and z. I can confidently say that I do not struggle daily with the thought of skipping meals. I do not mean to say that I am forever immune to having an ED again, but I am aware that this has been an issue for me in the past and since I may be prone to relapse, I do not own a scale, I don't spend more time looking in the mirror than I need to, and I eat even when I don't feel like it. These are things my husband, for example, doesn't need to think about, but I consciously make little decisions like these to keep me out of temptation's way. This is not a struggle. I do not agonize over these choices. I have tasted freedom (and chocolate) and will continue to safeguard my life so that a relapse is highly unlikely.

The temptations in your life are no different from what others experience. And God is faithful. He will not allow the temptation to be more than you can stand. When you are tempted, He will show you a way out so that you can endure (1 Corinthians 10:13).

So humble yourselves before God. Resist the devil, and he will flee from you (James 4:7).

Absolutely admit when you are currently struggling. This whole idea is not to shame anyone when she isn't able to handle addiction or disorder on her own. My plea is only to be careful with your words so that you don't trap yourself into just waiting for the relapse once you've become too tired to carry on in battle. I just hate the sense of doom that comes with the idea of always struggling.

There are two things in my life that I am currently struggling with: migraines and depression. If I believed I would have to constantly do battle with these issues for the rest of my life, I'd want to throw in the towel now. I have had those temptations when I thought this was never going to end. Unfortunately, we see that happening far too often. And so I am seeking help—coping mechanisms, support systems, correct treatments—until I can get over the hump and into recovery. Only then can I live a life safeguarding myself from relapses rather than just waiting things out until they get bad again.

Safeguarding your sobriety and health will require that you can honestly identify the triggers in your life and then do everything you can to flee from those temptations. As promised above, God will show you a way out.

For I can do everything through Christ, who gives me strength (Philippians 4:13).

I know there are plenty of you who are currently dealing with something very difficult. You might be wondering what's the point in getting help if you're going to have to fight against this all your life? You might think it's easier to just give in. This is why we need to stop claiming permanent bondage to our current struggle. Get the recovery you need, and then live your life in a way that keeps you safe and/or distant from triggers (support systems, therapy, nutrition and exercise, new friends, deeper bible study, etc.). The first few months or so may be tough, but once you've found your footing you'll be dancing in your freedom for years to come.

*

My mission in life is not merely to survive, but
to thrive; and to do so with some passion, some
compassion, some humor, and some style.
MAYA ANGELOU

*

CHAPTER TWENTY

Meet the writers

No act of kindness,
no matter how small,
is ever wasted.
AESOP

*

*

JUNE ALEXANDER
June is a 65-year-old living beyond anorexia nervosa
www.junealexander.com

June Alexander is a grandmother, writer, and international award-winning advocate in the field of eating disorders. She developed anorexia nervosa at age eleven in 1962, an illness which has largely shaped her life. Today June is a non-fiction storyteller, with a special passion for the diary. Her latest title, *Using Writing as a Therapy for Eating Disorders—The Diary Healer*, is the main component in her Ph.D. in Creative Writing.

June resigned from a longtime career in print journalism in 2007 to write her memoir, *A Girl Called Tim—Escape From An Eating Disorder Hell*. This sharing of her inner story led to the writing of more books about eating disorders, both for health practitioners and mainstream readers. June enjoys presenting life-writing workshops to people of all ages, and believes everyone has a story to tell. Involved in eating disorder advocacy at local, national and international level, June lives in Melbourne, Australia. Her family comprises four children and five grandchildren who are her best "medicine" and are experts at ensuring she lives in the moment.

Book titles with Routledge
London Taylor and Francis
Publishing Group
http://bit.ly/1TQqBv2

Ed Says U Said, Jessica Kingsley
Publishers
http://bit.ly/1tplkm1

A Girl Called Tim, Dennis Jones
http://bit.ly/SOpcKC

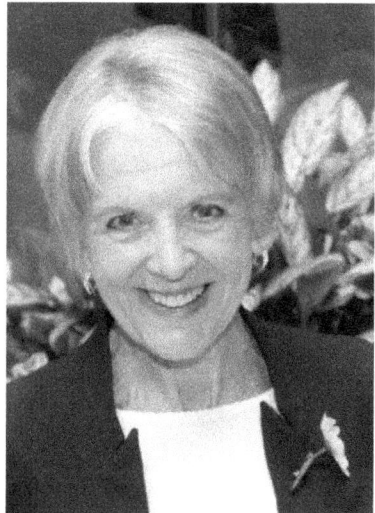

*

OLIVIA ANTHONY
Olivia is a 44-year-old living
with anorexia and bulimia
oliviaanthony1971@gmail.com

Olivia Anthony grew up in Billings, Montana. She earned her B. A. in Psychology from Concordia College in Moorhead, Minnesota. She lives with her husband, two children, and three cats in Seattle, Washington. She loves walking and bicycling in nature, reading, and do-it-yourself projects. She is working on finishing a book about her healing journey.

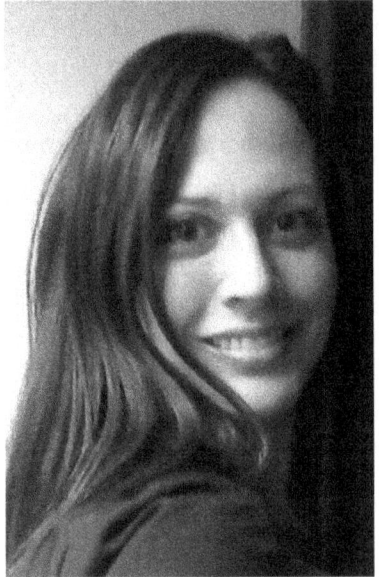

*

CHRISTINE BASTONE
Christine is a 49-year-old living
with binge eating disorder
C.Bastone@mail.com * www.facebook.com/CricketsPlace1

Christine Bastone is a stay-at-home mom in her forties who has only recently figured out that she wants to be a writer when she grows up! She was born in northeast Ohio, and moved to Florida in May 1995. She married Angelo Bastone in July 1997. They have a son, Joshua, born in 2001, and a daughter, Katelyn, born in 2004. The four of them live at the end of a quiet street in central Florida. Christine has always loved to read, and was thrilled when her husband gave her a Kindle for Christmas in 2011. She has since read hundreds of Kindle books.

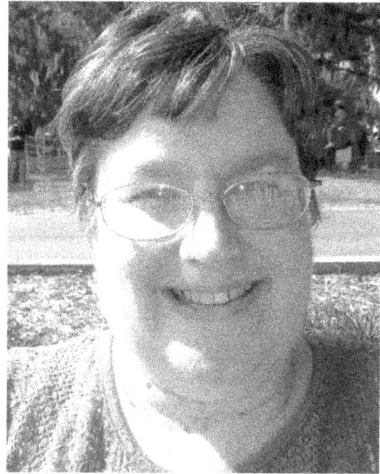

Christine is an award-winning writer of *Grief Diaries: Surviving Loss by Suicide*, coauthor of *Grief Diaries: Surviving Loss of a Sibling,* and has contributed to a number of books in the Grief Diaries and Real Life Diaries series. She has also been a guest on Grief Diaries Radio twice in 2014; both episodes are available on iTunes. At the time of this publication she is working on a new book called *Advice from Tomorrow.*

*

LISA BRUNS
Lisa is a 52-year-old living
with binge eating disorder

Lisa Bruns was born in Kaufman, Texas, to a white mother and Hispanic father. She graduated in 1982. She was very obese until age twenty-four, when she lost seventy pounds on her own, and then her doctor prescribed diet pills. At the age of forty-eight, Lisa underwent gastric bypass and lost one hundred pounds, but has since gained back eighty.

*

LYNDA CHELDELIN FELL
Lynda is a 50-year-old living
with binge eating disorder

Lynda Cheldelin Fell is an international best-selling author who is dedicated to helping people share their stories.

She is the creator of the award-winning Grief Diaries and Real Life Diaries book series, and CEO of AlyBlue Media.

A mother and grandmother, she resides in the beautiful Pacific Northwest with her family.

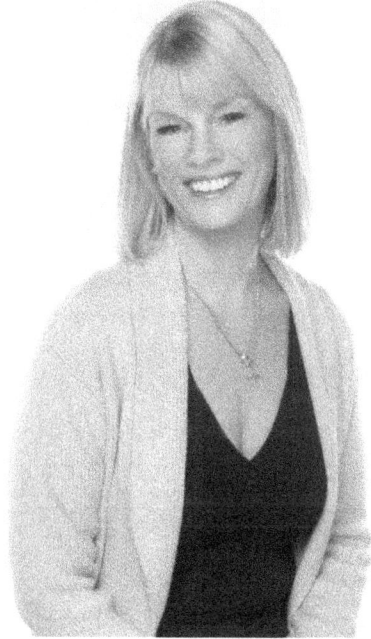

*

JUSTINE HILDEN
Justine is a 27-year-old living
with binge eating disorder

Justine was raised in East Bethel, Minnesota, with her mom, dad, and younger brother. She graduated with her B.A. in Elementary Education from Bethel University. Finding a passion in working with children with special needs, Justine went on to get a M.S. in Special Education from St. Cloud State University.

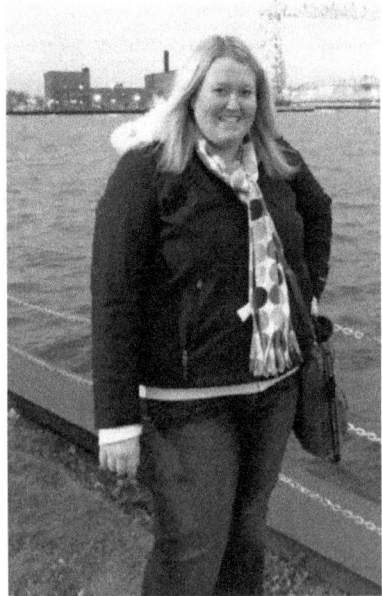

Justine is currently a teacher in a level IV special education program, teaching students with autism and emotional behavioral disorders.

When she is not working, she likes to spend time with her pets, friends, and family.

*

LYDIA KENYON
Lydia is a 22-year-old living
with anorexia nervosa

Lydia is a wife, daughter, friend and barista in a small town in Iowa. She spends her time making delicious coffee drinks, reading in every spare moment, and recovering from anorexia through treatment and blogging.

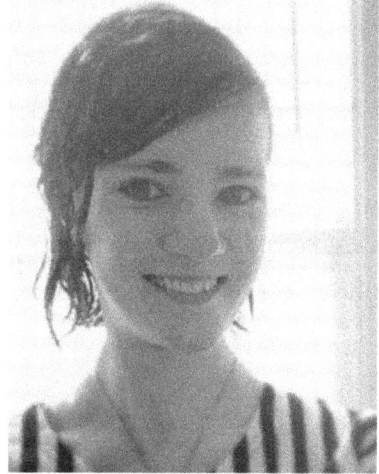

*

REBEKKAH KOONS
Rebekkah is a 29-year-old living with
an eating disorder not otherwise specified

Rebekkah Jane Koons is from the small town of Keene, New Hampshire, and currently works at her local hospital. In her spare time, she writes young adult book reviews, freelances for the local ad paper, and hopes to be volunteering with the local YMCA's gymnastics team. Rebekkah is currently working on her Bachelor's Degree in Literature and for down time enjoys hanging out with her Shih Tzu, Haddy.

*

MONICA MIRKES
Monica is a 58-year-old living
with binge eating disorder
monica.mirkes@yahoo.com

Monica Mirkes was born and raised in Texas. She had four children, two boys and two girls, and juggled all the "mom" jobs including carpools, Boy Scout den leader, Camp Fire leader, church, pets, and home. She did this with endless energy and humor. Through it all she cared for a medically fragile child. Monica could always find a way to make you laugh no matter what you were doing.

After raising her own children, Monica found herself working with preschoolers, which led to her becoming a Montessori teacher. Her gift for making each child feel special, along with their families, makes her a very special person.

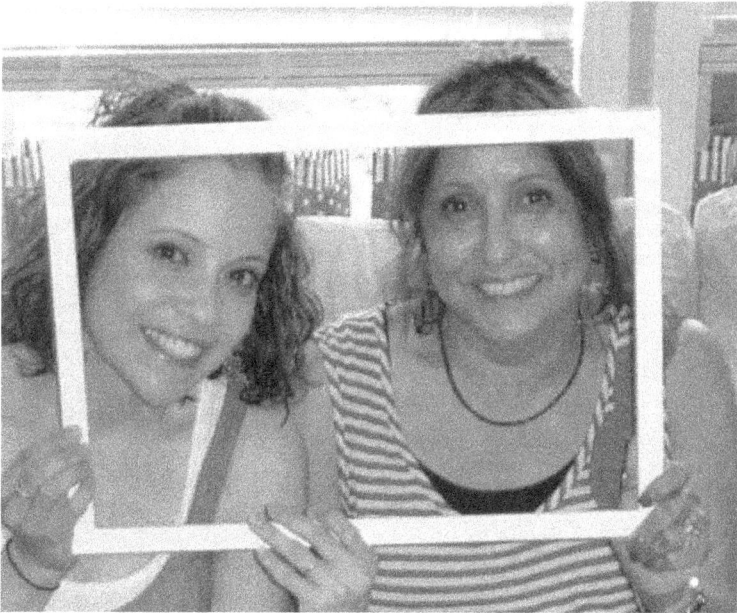

*

RUTH PAPALAS
Ruth is a 58-year-old living
with binge eating disorder

Ruth Papalas was born and raised in northeast Ohio, and earned a Business Administration degree in 1999. Her career includes working for several restaurants and housing authorities in Ohio. Ruth recently relocated and now resides with her retired husband in South Carolina, near her son and daughter-in-law. She also has a daughter, son-in-law and grandson who live in Ohio. She loves to spend time with her family, friends and dogs. She enjoys going to garage sales and locating unique items. She loves to travel, especially to Jamaica.

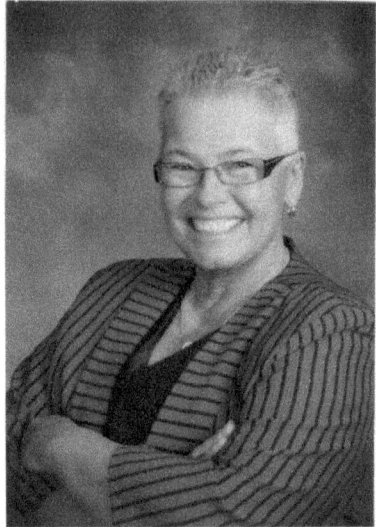

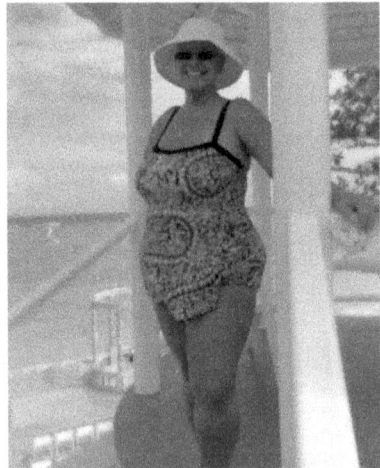

Since relocating to South Carolina, Ruth met new friends including Mary Lee Robinson, whom Ruth assisted in the writing of *The Widow or Widower Next Door.* Ruth is a contributor to the Grief Diaries series, having shared her story in *Grief Diaries: Surviving Loss of a Parent.*

*

DEBBIE PFIFFNER
Debbie is a 56-year-old living
with anorexia nervosa

Debbie Pfiffner was born and raised in St. Paul, Minnesota, the youngest of four girls. There she attended thirteen years of private school.

She worked as a public records researcher, which enabled her to travel extensively, especially in the Pacific Northwest, before leaving her job in 2007 to pursue other interests. Debbie also holds a manicurist's license, although she does not hold a position in that field.

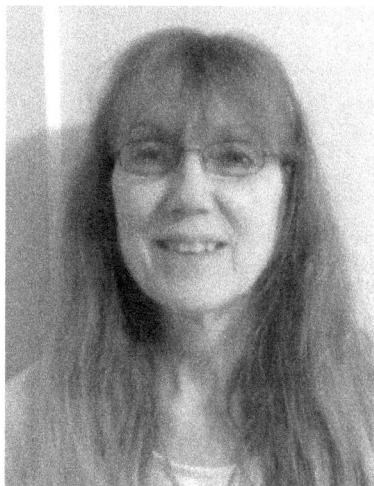

She was single and planned to remain so until she met her future husband. They married when Debbie was forty-seven years old. She has no children, but has had various "fur babies" throughout the years. Debbie is at present a homemaker, and she and her husband currently reside in her hometown of St. Paul. Her hobbies include reading, learning new things, knitting, and beading. On any given weekend during the NASCAR season you will find Debbie watching the NASCAR Sprint Cup Series and cheering for her favorite NASCAR driver, Tony Stewart.

*

DENISE PURCELL
Denise is a 50-year-old living
with anorexia nervosa and bulimia

Denise Purcell was born and raised in Syracuse, New York. She is the mother of four surviving girls. Denise is a strong advocate for many injustices that she herself has overcome. She is striving to make her dreams come true with her art and writing, and inspires others to do the same. Her youngest daughter is now in college, and starting her own journey in life.

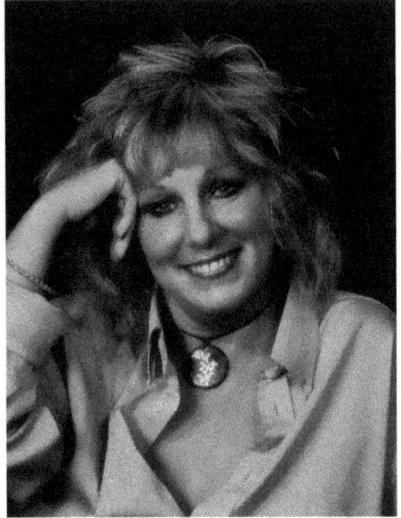

A prolific writer, Denise authored and illustrated Color My Soul Whole, coauthored Real Life Diaries: Through the Eyes of DID, and her work has been published in numerous Grief Diaries and Real Life Diaries titles. Sunshine has her own YouTube series, Sister Diaries with Sunshine, to raise awareness about living with DID.

Learn more at www.sisterdiarieswithsunshine.com.

*

HADDI TREBISOVSKY
Haddi is a 29-year-old living
with anorexia nervosa

Haddi Trebisovsky earned her B.A. in Elementary Education at Bethel University in St. Paul, Minnesota. She worked as a behavioral therapist for children with autism before leaving the workforce to be a stay-at-home mom to her two children. She enjoys writing and does so in the hope that it will bring encouragement and freedom to her readers. She is passionate about seeking the truth, and believes that the battles we face are more than just physical or mental, but also spiritual, and she brings this perspective forward in her experience with eating disorders, anxiety, depression, and suicidal thoughts.

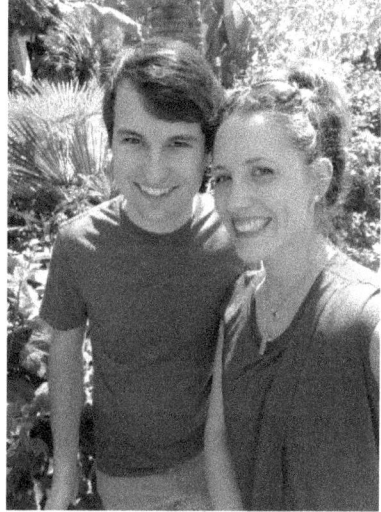

One smile can change a day.
One hug can change a life
One hope can change a destiny.
LYNDA CHELDELIN FELL

*

Thank you

I am deeply indebted to the writers of this book. It requires tremendous courage to bare such vulnerability about a topic so misunderstood. The individual dedication to seeing this project to the end is a legacy to be proud of. I'm especially grateful to coauthors June Alexander and Debbie Pfiffner, two ladies I admire immensely for their dedication to raise awareness about living with eating disorders. With very little nonclinical information available, it is my sincere hope that readers who share the same path will find compassion and hope, family and friends will gain better understanding, and professionals will appreciate the candid insight.

Helen Keller once said, "Walking with a friend in the dark is better than walking alone in the light." By sharing our struggles, we learn that we aren't truly alone as we travel our journey, for there are others ahead of us and some behind us. That is what Real Life Diaries is all about.

Lynda Cheldelin Fell xoxo

Shared joy is doubled joy;
shared sorrow is half a sorrow.
SWEDISH PROVERB

*

ABOUT

Lynda Cheldelin Fell

Considered a pioneer in the field of inspirational hope in the aftermath of hardship and loss, Lynda Cheldelin Fell has a passion for storytelling and producing groundbreaking projects that create a legacy of help, healing, and hope.

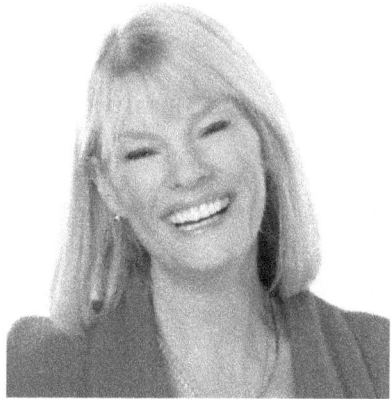

She is an international best-selling author and creator of the award-winning book series Grief Diaries and Real Life Diaries. Her repertoire of interviews include Dr. Martin Luther King's daughter, Trayvon Martin's mother, sisters of the late Nicole Brown Simpson, Pastor Todd Burpo of Heaven Is For Real, CNN commentator Dr. Ken Druck, and other societal newsmakers on finding healing and hope in the aftermath of life's harshest challenges.

Lynda's own story began in 2007, when she had an alarming dream about her young teenage daughter, Aly. In the dream, Aly was a backseat passenger in a car that veered off the road and landed in a lake. Aly sank with the car, leaving behind an open book floating face down on the water. Two years later, Lynda's dream became reality when her daughter was killed as a backseat passenger in a car accident while coming home from a swim meet. Overcome with grief, Lynda's forty-six-year-old husband suffered a major stroke that left him with severe disabilities, changing the family dynamics once again.

The following year, Lynda was invited to share her remarkable story about finding hope after loss, and she accepted. That cathartic experience inspired her to create groundbreaking projects spanning national events, radio, film and books to help others who share the same journey feel less alone. Now a passionate curator of stories, Lynda is dedicated to helping ordinary people share their own extraordinary journeys that touch the hearts of both reader and writer.

lynda@lyndafell.com | www.lyndafell.com

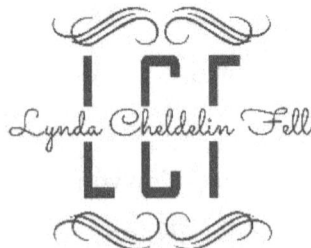

ALYBLUE MEDIA TITLES

Real Life Diaries: Living with Mental Illness
Real Life Diaries: Living with Endometriosis
Real Life Diaries: Living with Rheumatic Disease
Real Life Diaries: Living with a Brain Injury
Real Life Diaries: Through the Eyes of DID
Real Life Diaries: Through the Eyes of an Eating Disorder
Grief Diaries: Surviving Loss of a Spouse
Grief Diaries: Surviving Loss of a Child
Grief Diaries: Surviving Loss of a Sibling
Grief Diaries: Surviving Loss of a Parent
Grief Diaries: Surviving Loss of an Infant
Grief Diaries: Surviving Loss of a Loved One
Grief Diaries: Surviving Loss by Suicide
Grief Diaries: Surviving Loss of Health
Grief Diaries: How to Help the Newly Bereaved
Grief Diaries: Loss by Impaired Driving
Grief Diaries: Loss by Homicide
Grief Diaries: Loss of a Pregnancy
Grief Diaries: Hello from Heaven
Grief Diaries: Grieving for the Living
Grief Diaries: Shattered
Grief Diaries: Project Cold Case
Grief Diaries: Poetry & Prose and More
Grief Diaries: Through the Eyes of Men
Grief Diaries: Will We Survive?
Grief Diaries: Hit by Impaired Driver
Grammy Visits From Heaven
Grandpa Visits From Heaven
Faith, Grief & Pass the Chocolate Pudding
Heaven Talks to Children
God's Gift of Love: After Death Communication
Color My Soul Whole
Grief Reiki

To share your story, visit
www.griefdiaries.com
www.RealLifeDiaries.com

PUBLISHED BY ALYBLUE MEDIA
Inside every human is a story worth sharing.
www.AlyBlueMedia.com

AlyBlue
MEDIA

www.ingramcontent.com/pod-product-compliance
Lightning Source LLC
Chambersburg PA
CBHW031140020426
42333CB00013B/451